T0382949

4D Imaging to 4D Printing

This book focuses on applications of 4D imaging and 4D printing for development of low-cost, indigenous lab-scale solutions for various biomedical applications. It is based on a selection of benchmark open-source 4D imaging solutions including the effect of different stimulus (such as light, electric field, magnetic field, mechanical load, thermal, hydro, and so forth) to better understand the 4D capabilities of printed components. The material is covered across nine chapters dedicated to 4D imaging, 4D printing, and their specific biomedical applications illustrated via case studies related to the orthopedic and dental requirements of veterinary patients.

The book:

- Presents exclusive material on the integration of 4D imaging and 4D printing
- Demonstrates the industrial applications of 4D imaging in 4D printing using multiple case studies
- Discusses use of open-source 4D imaging tools for biomedical applications
- Includes in-house development of smart materials for 4D printing
- Reviews low-cost, indigenous lab-scale solutions for various veterinary applications.

This book is aimed at graduate students and researchers in Additive Manufacturing, Manufacturing Engineering, Production Engineering, Mechanical Engineering, and Materials Engineering.

Emerging Materials and Technologies

Series Editor: Boris I. Kharissov

The *Emerging Materials and Technologies* series is devoted to highlighting publications centered on emerging advanced materials and novel technologies. Attention is paid to those newly discovered or applied materials with potential to solve pressing societal problems and improve quality of life, corresponding to environmental protection, medicine, communications, energy, transportation, advanced manufacturing, and related areas.

The series takes into account that, under present strong demands for energy, material, and cost savings, as well as heavy contamination problems and worldwide pandemic conditions, the area of emerging materials and related scalable technologies is a highly interdisciplinary field, with the need for researchers, professionals, and academics across the spectrum of engineering and technological disciplines. The main objective of this book series is to attract more attention to these materials and technologies and invite conversation among the international R&D community.

Emerging Nanomaterials for Catalysis and Sensor Applications
Edited by Anitha Varghese and Gurumurthy Hegde

Advanced Materials for a Sustainable Environment
Development Strategies and Applications
Edited by Naveen Kumar and Peter Ramashadi Makgwane

Nanomaterials from Renewable Resources for Emerging Applications
Edited by Sandeep S. Ahankari, Amar K. Mohanty, and Manjusri Misra

Multifunctional Polymeric Foams
Advancements and Innovative Approaches
Edited by Soney C George and Resmi B. P.

Nanotechnology Platforms for Antiviral Challenges
Fundamentals, Applications and Advances
Edited by Soney C George and Ann Rose Abraham

Carbon-Based Conductive Polymer Composites
Processing, Properties, and Applications in Flexible Strain Sensors
Dong Xiang

Nanocarbons
Preparation, Assessments, and Applications
Ashwini P. Alegaonkar and Prashant S. Alegaonka

4D Imaging to 4D Printing
Biomedical Applications
Edited by Rupinder Singh

For more information about this series, please visit: www.routledge.com/Emerging-Materials-and-Technologies/book-series/CRCEMT

4D Imaging to 4D Printing

Biomedical Applications

Edited by
Rupinder Singh

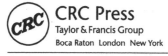

CRC Press
Taylor & Francis Group
Boca Raton London New York

CRC Press is an imprint of the
Taylor & Francis Group, an **informa** business

Cover image: ©Shutterstock

First edition published 2023
by CRC Press
6000 Broken Sound Parkway NW, Suite 300, Boca Raton, FL 33487-2742

and by CRC Press
4 Park Square, Milton Park, Abingdon, Oxon, OX14 4RN

CRC Press is an imprint of Taylor & Francis Group, LLC

ISBN: 9781032071367 (hbk)
ISBN: 9781032071381 (pbk)
ISBN: 9781003205531 (ebk)

DOI: 10.1201/9781003205531

Typeset in Times
by Deanta Global Publishing Services, Chennai, India

Contents

Editor Biography

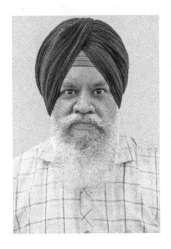

Dr. Rupinder Singh is a Professor in the Department of Mechanical Engineering, National Institute of Technical Teacher Training and Research, Chandigarh. He has received a PhD in Mechanical Engineering from the Thapar Institute of Engineering and Technology Patiala. His area of research is additive manufacturing, composite filament processing, rapid tooling, metal casting, and plastic solid waste management. He has co-authored more than 350 science citation-indexed research papers, 10 books, and more than 150 book chapters, and has presented more than 100 research papers in various national/international journals. His research has been cited more than 10,210 times with an H index of 47 and a Google Scholar i-10 index of 212. As per Stanford University, he has been listed among the world's top 2% scientists.

Contributors

Inderpreet Singh Ahuja
Dept. of Mechanical Engineering,
Punjabi University, Patiala
(Punjab, India).

Sukhwant Singh Banwait
Dept. of Mechanical Engineering,
National Institute of Technical
Teacher Training and Research,
Chandigarh.

Abhishek Barwar
Dept. of Mechanical Engineering,
National Institute of Technical
Teacher Training and Research,
Chandigarh.

Kamaljit Singh Boparai
Dept. of Mechanical Engineering,
Giani Zail Singh Campus College
of Engineering and Technology,
Bathinda, India.

Anish Das
Dept. of Mechanical Engineering,
National Institute of Technical
Teacher Training and Research,
Chandigarh.

Minhaz Husain
Dept. of Mechanical Engineering,
National Institute of Technical
Teacher Training and Research,
Chandigarh.

Deepika Kathuria
Department of Mechanical
Engineering and University Centre
for Research and Development,
Chandigarh University, Punjab,
India.

Abhishek Kumar
Dept. of Mechanical Engineering,
National Institute of Technical
Teacher Training and Research,
Chandigarh.

Ranvijay Kumar
University Centre for Research
and Development, Chandigarh
University, Mohali (India),
Department of Mechanical
Engineering, National Institute of
Technical Teachers Training and
Research, Chandigarh.

Vinay Kumar
Dept. of Mechanical and Production
Engineering, Guru Nanak Dev
Engineering College, Ludhiana
Punjab, India, and University Center
for Research and Development,
Chandigarh University, Mohali.

Smruti Ranjan Pradhan
Dept. of Mechanical Engineering,
National Institute of Technical
Teacher Training and Research,
Chandigarh.

Nishant Ranjan
Dept. of Mechanical Engineering and
University Centre for Research
and Development, Chandigarh
University, Punjab, India.

Vaibhav Sahani
Senior Project Research Fellow, Unit of
Periodontics, Oral Health Sciences
Centre, Post Graduate Institute of
Medical Education and Research
Chandigarh.

Ajay Sharma
Dept. of Mechanical Engineering and
    University Centre for Research
    and Development, Chandigarh
    University, Punjab, India.

Rupinder Singh
Dept. of Mechanical Engineering,
    National Institute of Technical
    Teacher Training and Research,
    Chandigarh.

Preface

4D Imaging to 4D Printing: Biomedical Applications aims to present comprehensively the most recent breakthroughs in the use of 4D imaging and 4D printing for biomedical applications. The book delivers an optimized and fool-proofed methodology of using 4D imaging and 4D printing, keeping in view the need for biomedical application (for academic researchers as well as field practitioners). Overall, the book focuses on the application of 4D imaging and 4D printing for the development of low-cost, indigenous lab-scale solutions for various biomedical applications.

The book highlights the integration of 4D imaging and 4D printing, the use of open-source 4D imaging tools for biomedical applications, orthopedic and dental 4D requirements for veterinary patients, and low-cost, indigenous lab-scale solutions for various biomedical applications of veterinary patients: clinical dentistry and orthopedics; in-house development of smart materials for 4D printing. Also outlined are: case studies on dentistry applications using medical imaging; the use of in-house prepared filament for 4D printing applications in orthopedics; 4D-imaging-assisted 4D printing for clinical dentistry of canines; 4D-imaging-assisted 4D printing for an efficient drug delivery system for veterinary cancer patients.

Overall, this book is a first-hand source of information for academic scholars and field engineers for preoperative strategic planning.

Dr. Rupinder Singh
Chandigarh (India)

1 Integration of 4D Imaging with 4D Printing

Kamaljit Singh Boparai, Abhishek Kumar, and Rupinder Singh

CONTENTS

1.1 INTRODUCTION

In a three-dimensional (3D) coordination system, each axis points in an independent direction and creates a 3D space. Usually, the fourth dimension is represented by an amount of time. The reality of human beings is specified by the three spatial dimensions and time is an additional, temporary dimension that moves in a single direction, from birth until death. These four dimensions can be understood and even visualized. However, the fourth dimension can also be about looking at something much less intuitive and much more complex, where time is not being considered as a fourth spatial dimension – a dimension that cannot be touched, seen, or even entered into, but at the same time exists all around us. To understand this, first consider a two-dimensional (2D) plane called a flatland: a place inhabited by two-dimensional creatures. These creatures (called flatlanders) exist entirely within two dimensions (X and Y spaces) and, for them, there is no Z-axis (no third dimension). Similarly, 3D objects have three dimensions along the X-, Y-, and Z-axes respectively. In flatland,

DOI: 10.1201/9781003205531-1

1

it is possible to move them left or right, forward or backward, but moving in a new direction would be moving out of reality, which is impossible. So, travel to the fourth dimension requires moving somewhere else, somewhere that's perpendicular to all three of these directions (thus, inward or outward). These directions mean nothing, but they exist in a four-dimensional (4D) world. Without physically going into the fourth dimension, it is possible to visualize the world from the 4D point of view. Since the flatlander lives in a two-dimensional plane, the one-dimensional (1D) projection of the shapes is visualized e.g., a circle on a flatland looks like a line. When the circle moves toward them, the line grows and when it moves away it appears to shrink. As the flatlander can only be illustrated as lines, its real shape and its distinction from another flatlander may appear confusing, but it is quite simple. Not only do the flatlanders have depth perception but flat layers also have other senses they can feel by touching the size of objects. A flatlander can figure out how these lines come together by the shape they make. It is possible to study a shape from different angles. Generally, the eye can see 2D projections of our 3D world. We only see shapes through our senses, but we can recognize how these shapes come together and form 3D objects. We can recognize a cube just by looking at it from a single angle.

A flatland plane sees lines that make shapes, and the eye sees shapes that make up 3D objects; therefore, a 4D creature would see 3D objects that make hyper objects. So, looking at the world through the fourth dimension, we would see the entirety of our world, just as we can see the entirety of the flatland plane. In other words, where the flatland plane only sees one side of a square, we see the entire square. On the other hand, we see only one side of a cube, but if we looked at the same cube from the fourth dimension, it would be possible to see the whole cube with its six sides simultaneously. Thinking in higher dimensions is difficult, although it can be done, but how can we study the fourth dimension if we cannot physically see it? How can it possibly be understood? This can be imagined by how a flatlander learns about our world. In a flatland, the circle can be specified in two dimensions (XY). The circle can move up or down, right or left, but it is restricted in a plane XY of flatland. Now imagine that a circle looks as if its diameter is shrinking to a tiny point and disappearing and growing back to its original size. It is not a circle; it is a projection of the sphere on flatland associated with the direction of up and down. When 3D objects intersect a flatland, the projections of a cross section of the object can be moved up or down, left or right as objects move in the XY plane, but it also moves perpendicular to the plane (forward or backward). It is possible to form a sphere with these projections. In this manner, it is possible to imagine the shape of an object with the projections on flatland. It is also possible to picture the higher-dimension geometry with little information by considering the lower-dimension projections of the 3D objects and the direction in which the object is moving. In this manner, it is possible to build a mental image of the object through a compilation of the visible slices (projections). Similarly, when a 4D object passes through the flatland plane, instead of 2D slices, 3D slices of 4D objects appear. So, 3D projections appear to change as they move perpendicular to the flatland plane.

In reality, we are looking at the 3D objects or slices of 4D objects as they pass through the hyperplane. By studying these slices, it is possible to build an understanding of the geometry of 4D objects. In mathematics, a circle (2D object) can be represented by Equation 1.1.

$$x^2 + y^2 = r^2$$ (Equation 1.1)

As per Equation 1, it is possible to change the circle's size and location by changing its coordinates.

However, a sphere (3D object) can be represented by Equation 1.2. In this case, the additional z dimension is added.

$$x^2 + y^2 + z^2 = r^2$$ (Equation 1.2)

In 4D, this can be visualized by adding one more dimension (w), to transfer a sphere into a 4D object called a 4D hypersphere, and Equation 1.3 can be used to determine the shape of 3D slices. If this hypersphere has to pass through the hyperplane (in this case, it is a world), the equation is reduced to Equation 1.4.

$$x^2 + y^2 + z^2 + w^2 = r^2$$ (Equation 1.3)

$$x^2 + y^2 + z^2 = r^2 - w^2$$ (Equation 1.4)

Equation 4 becomes the equation of a sphere, which means that 3D slices of the hyperplane are spheres, and the size of the spherical slices depends upon the hyperplane not upon coordinates, as shown in Figure 1.1.

When a 3D sphere intersects flatland, it creates a growing and shrinking circle, caused by the roundness of the sphere in three dimensions. Flatlander can compile these slices and visualize their 3D roundness by observing the rate of change of the radius. Similarly, as the hypersphere moves through the hyperplane, it shows the sphere can grow and shrink according to curvature in the fourth dimension.

1.2 4D IMAGING

The advent of 4D imaging introduced advanced image vision that provides an object's state-of-the-art, real-time function at the micro and macro levels. It was the

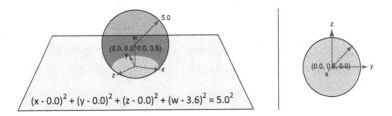

FIGURE 1.1   4D hypersphere.

need for the time-lapse study of living objects that brought about 4D imaging. The first time-lapse electronic timer was developed in 1960 and was capable of controlling the shutter at predetermined intervals and staging movement so that deeper information can be extracted from different focal planes (Gustafson and Kinnander, 1960). It should be noted that by 1985 all the digital systems required for 4D data-set acquisition had been developed and existed in a basic form (Turano et al., 1985). The term "4D imaging" is used to describe the three-dimensional imaging space that varies with the dynamic change of elements over time; 4D imaging is merely 3D imaging with the dynamic feature. In 4D imaging, 2D or 3D images are first captured from inaccessible locations with laser, radiation, sonography, or tomography; 4D imaging is an advanced image analysis method that combines slices of 3D imaging with the time cycle in such a way that movement and any variation in movement can be observed more accurately and precisely (Kanaga et al., 2021). It increases the understanding of a process by providing detailed image information concerning time which assists in faster image interpretation and reduction in significant errors of movement, which is the main challenge in 3D imaging. A 4D image data set consists of multiple sequentially stacked 3D image data sets at subsequent time points which highlights the state of the process over time. The captured data is then image-processed with inbuilt algorithms to generate 4D images. The rapid growth in hardware and software packages of image acquisition and processing has made visualizing the interior detail of an object in a dynamic environment and, more often, of the living subject, quite easy; these packages help in analyzing an object in numerous ways from different angles and on different focal planes (Thomas and White, 1998).

The basic 4D imaging data-acquisition hardware setup (shown in Figure 1.2) consists of the following components: magnifier, detector, motor drives, digitizer, and a computer system (Thomas and White, 1998).

(1) An imaging instrument (usually a magnifier or microscope) with high resolution, a correct optics system with image-sectioning capabilities, and apparatus for keeping the living organism alive while the experiment is being run.
(2) A detector (maybe a digital or analog camera) to record the movement of magnified images in the form of signals with accurate scanning functionalities.
(3) Motor drives that can be controlled with a computer system to move the imaging planes in the required direction.
(4) A digitizer to convert the detected signals into digital signals that are compatible with computer-friendly extensions.
(5) A computer system to store, view, analyze, and manipulate the acquired data set for 4D imaging.

The well-developed 4D imaging system should have basic functionalities to fully visualize, analyze, interpret, manipulate, and archive, dynamic 3D movements in computerized digital mode, to view 4D data as single-rendered 3D volume (Kriete

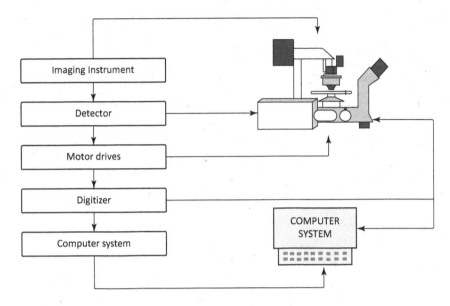

FIGURE 1.2   4D imaging system.

and Wagner, 1993), view 3D data slices as a reconstructed object (Errington et al., 1997) with motion analysis (Lin et al., 1996) or computer animation (Malinda et al., 1995), object location, volume, intensity, and distance (Loew et al., 1993). Technological advances in 4D imaging are rapidly emerging with the introduction of machine learning (ML), artificial intelligence (AI), virtual reality (VR), and augmented reality (AR) tools; these generate 4D data sets accurately, from the smallest microscopic biological specimen or geological scale specimen to material science which indicates positive future development (Thomas and White, 1998).

The conceptualization of four-dimensional imaging began with the use of ultrasound in prenatal clinics which allowed parents to observe, in stacks of 3D images, the behavior of the unborn baby and for care and abnormalities to be checked. The applications of 4D imaging (shown in Figure 1.3) are not limited to clinical studies but find application in Industry 4.0, Health 4.0, Agriculture 4.0, autonomous vehicles, or ADAS (advanced driver-assistance systems), remote sensing, material microscopy, disaster management, and 4D imaging radar.

1.3   INTEGRATION OF 4D IMAGING WITH 4D PRINTING

The area of 4D printing with 4D imaging is not much explored and it should be noted that exploration of 4D space in 3D printing has a wide range of applications in various sectors that can be integrated with 4D imaging, ranging from the development of assistive tool production in the medical, manufacturing, agriculture fields to cell-derived tissues or bioprinting of organs. The integration of 4D imaging with 4D printing could revolutionize product development process. 4D imaging can record the real-time function of a subject and with 4D printing, one can develop highly versatile

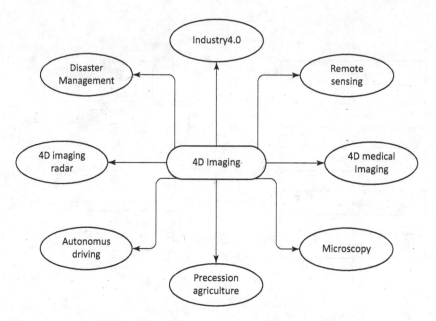

FIGURE 1.3 Applications of 4D imaging.

interdisciplinary applications, in medicine, in the field of soft robots, wearable electronics in the form of smart textiles, and other industries such as precision agriculture and the science of microfluidics. Developments in additive manufacturing (AM) and imaging have changed the dynamics of several industries, particularly medical and material science. 4D imaging has made it possible to record interior and exterior detail on different focal planes with real-time functions, eliminating the uncertainties associated with the voluntary and involuntary dynamic movement of the subject. 4D printing has provided an excellent opportunity for researchers and scientists to fabricate objects that can adapt to external stimuli over time; 4D capabilities may be reversible or irreversible under the effects of stimuli such as heat, load, solvents, and light. The integration of 4D imaging with 4D printing has provided an exciting opportunity to mimic real processes or extract the details of newly fabricated 4D-capable AM objects by using 4D imaging under the action of external response. Nowadays, 4D medical imaging data, especially that of four-dimensional computed tomography (4DCT) and four-dimensional magnetic resonance imaging (4DMRI), has made it possible to mimic the real-time formation of artificial implants which can be integrated into the body and which have 4D capabilities, such as those of being self-absorbing, self-healing, and self-expanding, and are, for example, thermo-, chemo-, and photo-responsive.

Using the keywords "4D imaging with 4D printing", "4D printing in agriculture", 4D printing in biomedical", "4D printing in sensor", 4D printing in industry 4.0", "4D printing in automotive", and "4D printing with novel material", analysis of the online science research database for the years 1999 to 2022 has established that there is a gap in the research. These web database results were further segregated based

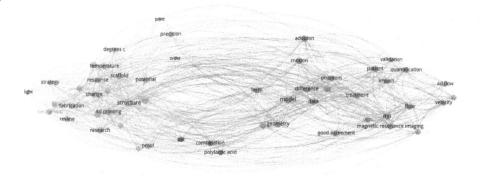

FIGURE 1.4 Bibliographic analysis for the keywords "4D imaging with 4D printing".

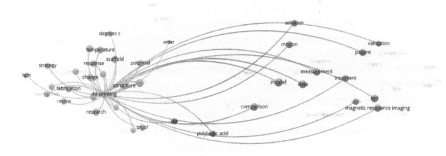

FIGURE 1.5 Research-gap analysis for "4D printing".

on the highest number of citations. In VOSviewer software used for the minimum number of occurrences of the term "5", 88 terms met the threshold out of 4,315 terms. Further for these 88 terms, a relevance score was calculated, and the top 60% of the term "53" were used for analysis (shown in Figures 1.4 to 1.19 and Table 1.1).

1.4 FUTURE TRENDS OF 4D IMAGING

1.4.1 AGRICULTURE 4.0

In the era of Agriculture 4.0, 4D imaging can provide farm managers with a precise crop monitoring system for knowing the status of crops for timely decision-making and early treatment of infected crops to avoid yield loss. It should be noted that as crops are constantly growing, changing color, and moving due to the wind, 4D imaging is essential for the study of dynamic nature because static 3D images cannot provide the required details for precision agriculture. The literature review reveals the use of unmanned aerial vehicles (UAV) or unmanned ground vehicles

TABLE 1.1
Relevance Score and Occurrences Data for Keywords "4D Imaging and 4D Printing"

S No.	Keyword	Occurrences	Relevance Score
1	4D flow	7	1.7018
2	4D printing	20	1.0921
3	Addition	9	0.4721
4	Aneurysm	9	1.3912
5	Architecture	13	1.2335
6	Cell	13	1.3995
7	Change	15	1.2261
8	Combination	5	0.1862
9	Comparison	12	0.2054
10	Concept	8	0.8196
11	Construct	9	2.1273
12	Data	27	0.3412
13	Degrees c	6	1.7829
14	Difference	14	0.5037
15	Fabrication	11	1.7933
16	Flow	20	1.2366
17	Formation	10	1.1902
18	Geometry	12	0.1339
19	Good agreement	5	0.7969
20	Hemodynamic	7	1.7555
21	Impact	6	1.2778
22	Light	6	2.1008
23	Magnetic resonance imaging	14	0.929
24	Measurement	19	0.653
25	Mechanism	12	1.3171
26	Model	31	0.3172
27	Motion	12	0.4683
28	MRI	18	1.1006
29	Order	5	0.4274
30	Patient	14	0.8571
31	Phantom	15	0.7724
32	PLA	6	0.7497
33	Polylactic acid	6	0.4127
34	Potential	11	0.5328
35	Precision	6	0.7365
36	Presence	5	0.9664
37	Print	5	1.1671
38	Proof	6	0.6364
39	Quantification	7	1.2982
40	Research	13	0.9649

(Continued)

TABLE 1.1 (CONTINUED)
**Relevance Score and Occurrences Data for Keywords
"4D Imaging and 4D Printing"**

S No.	Keyword	Occurrences	Relevance Score
41	Response	10	1.1217
42	Review	7	1.4476
43	Scaffold	10	1.3593
44	Shape	16	0.5874
45	Shape-memory polymer	7	1.3267
46	Strategy	10	1.8153
47	Structure	35	0.9045
48	Temperature	11	1.2946
49	Term	6	0.097
50	Treatment	8	0.7473
51	Validation	5	0.9867
52	Velocity	9	1.5658
53	Vitro	6	0.6718

(UGV), computer vision, and 4D image reconstruction while monitoring, spraying, weeding, or food picking (Nezhad et al., 2011; Siddiqi et al., 2009; Ried and Searcy, 1987).

The automatic guidance provided by the incorporation of 4D imaging in the tractor or ground vehicles in the agricultural field can reduce the mental fatigue of machine operators. Work on algorithms for computer vision for segmenting and crop guidance was first explored in 1991 (Ried and Searcy, 1991); work also took place on automatic tractor guidance for precision agriculture (Ried and Searcy, 1987). The literature review indicates the use of 4D reconstruction: estimates of the height and size of crops over time are made for precision agriculture by collecting multiple 3D image data for several weeks and by integrating sensor fusion and computer vision (Dong et al., 2014; Carlone et al., 2015). In the era of Agriculture 4.0, with the use of 4D imaging, we can make biophysical assessments and physiological evaluations, monitor biological targets, and spray bio-inputs and disinfectants to achieve increased productivity and reduce stress. 4D imaging data from the agriculture field can be extracted and can be used for 4D printing of fertilizer, food picking, weeding, etc.

1.4.2 IDENTIFICATION OF CROP SIZE AND GRADING

Computer-assisted crop-sorting or grading systems, in the case of precision agriculture, vary from product to product or even from product variety and size-wise. Work on the use of image processing to identify crop disease (Tian et al., 2011) has been highlighted, and similarly work on image processing to grade agriculture products

(Raj et al., 2015). A machine-vision system to classify plantlet segments of potatoes has been proposed by Alchanatis et al. (1993). The use of a machine-vision computer-mediated system to classify carrots based on surface defects, brokenness, and curvature has been reported (Haworth and Searcy, 1992). In economically backward countries it is done manually by labor or small-farm managers by themselves which increases the chance of significant human error (depending on physical and mental fitness) and consumes time. In manual sorting and grading, it is hard to maintain consistency and uniformity. To provide a solution to sorting and grading in precision agriculture a computer-assisted image-processing route can be mediated which can mimic the human sorting and grading of the crop with high accuracy and repeatability. There is a need, nowadays, for quality control in agriculture, due to adulteration and malpractice on the parts of traders using low-quality seed and fertilizers, which cannot be ignored, or is sometimes due to the biotic and abiotic environmental effect the crop quality degrades and lead to disease in crops. The bibliographic analysis for the keywords "agriculture additive manufacturing" and the research-gap analysis for "4D printing in agriculture" has been highlighted in Figures 1.6 and 1.7 respectively.

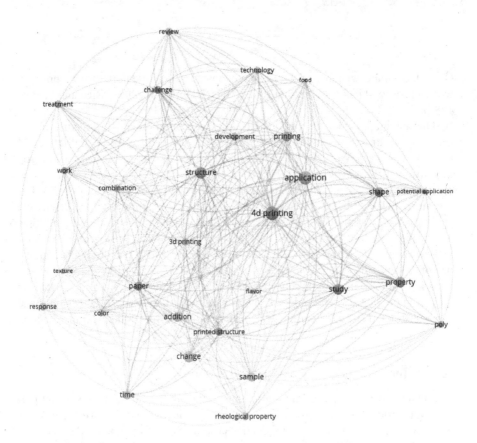

FIGURE 1.6 Bibliographic analysis for the keywords "agriculture additive manufacturing".

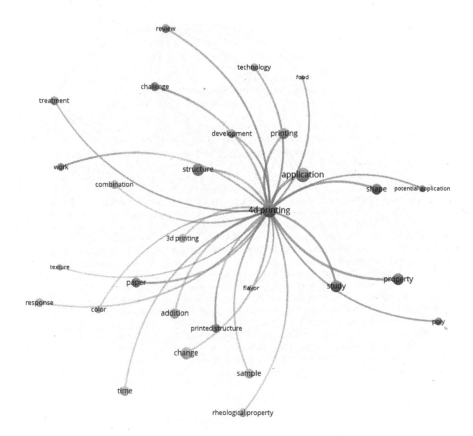

FIGURE 1.7 Research-gap analysis for "4D printing in agriculture".

1.4.3 INDUSTRY 4.0

Manufacturing industries and the industrial inspection sector are the latest to embrace 4D imaging for accurate part fabrication, quality checking, quality control, part inspection, and process-cycle defect recognition. The use of 4D imaging during the part manufacturing cycle on the shop floor can help managers monitor and optimize the operator workflow for industrial engineering method-study purposes. Installing a camera on the machine during the part fabrication process could help in situ identification of defective parts. The robotic and automation system in the industrial workplace nowadays uses cloud computing, artificial intelligence, machine learning, and big-data analytics to optimize the production process flow. The use of 4D imaging with the aforementioned technology can bring significant improvement in the industrial revolution and reduce mental stress in quality managers.

1.4.4 QUALITY CONTROL IN INDUSTRY BY IMAGING

Nowadays, competition between industries and technological advancement is rapidly booming due to the availability of highly precise mass customization machines and equipment. However, due to defective items being produced and lack of quality control and assurance, the reputation and standards of a company can be damaged, which can bring about loss of capital, a decrease in employee morale, and material wastage. Work on the use of infrared thermography to control quality on the production line has been reported (Grabowski and Cristalli, 2015). Similar work on the use of image processing to control manufacturing processes and compare the results with those obtained by human inspection has been outlined (Somwang and Muangklang, 2019). With the induction of automation and digitalization there is now automated visual inspection based on digital image processing and computer monitoring, which means that faulty parts can be detected and sorted out in the process. Digital image processing, deep learning, and machine-vision techniques can apply industry standards and measurements to identify defective parts. Bibliographic analysis for the keywords "4D printing in Industry 4.0" is shown in Figure 1.8 and analysis of the research gap for "4D food printing" and of shape-memory polymer is shown in Figures 1.9 and 1.10 respectively. The corresponding research gaps are shown in Figures 1.11 to 1.13.

1.4.5   HEALTH 4.0

Health care inspired by Industry 4.0 is known as Health 4.0, which is building a new paradigm for smart and connected health care (Li and Carayon, 2021). There are major applications of 4D medical imaging for recording and observing the movement

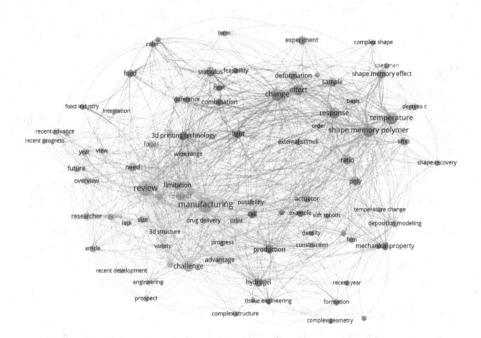

FIGURE 1.8   Bibliographic analysis for the keywords "4D printing in Industry 4.0 ".

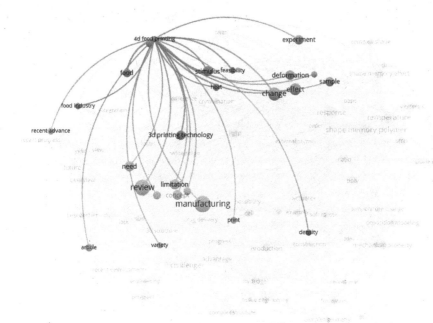

FIGURE 1.9   Research-gap analysis for "4D food printing".

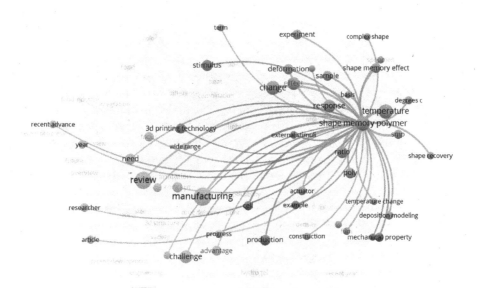

FIGURE 1.10   Research-gap analysis for "shape-memory polymer".

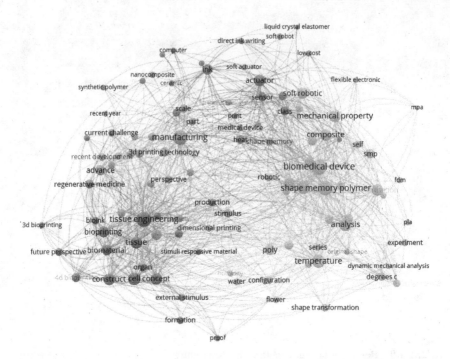

FIGURE 1.11   Bibliographic analysis for the keywords "4D printing in biomedical".

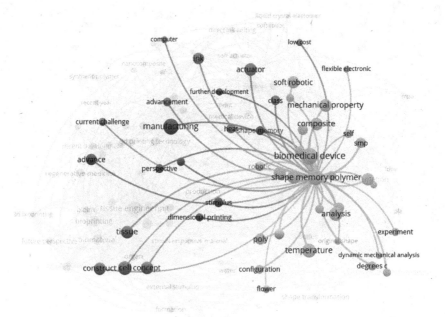

FIGURE 1.12   Research-gap analysis for "shape-memory polymer".

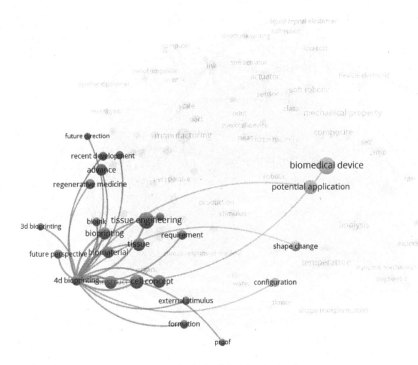

FIGURE 1.13   Research-gap analysis for "4D bioprinting".

per breath of a patient during advanced surgical procedures. The two basic elements of Health 4.0 are smartness and prediction analysis. It incorporates the use of artificial intelligence, big-data analytics, image processing, and machine learning for monitoring, optimal treatment, and intervention in the real-time care of the patient. The 4D imaging data in the health-care sector can assist surgeons in understanding the patient's breath cycle as the lungs inflate and deflate, dynamic movement of any organs, growth of a tumor, and the effect of movement of organs on a tumor. 4D medical imaging allows surgeons to design more precise preoperative surgical planning, resulting in reduced postoperative surgical complications and blood loss, and savings in surgical time. 4D medical imaging lends itself to the following modalities: computed tomography (CT), positron emission tomography (PET), magnetic resonance imaging (MRI), ultrasound (US) imaging, and single-photon emission computed tomography (SPECT), thus eliminating uncertainties and artifacts associated with patient's voluntary and involuntary organ movements, with the respiratory cycle, and with movement of the muscles (Li et al., 2008).

Due to its rapid image acquisition, diversified imaging mode, and improved image quality, 4D medical imaging is becoming more clinically applicable. In a 4D CT scan, a special CT scan machine is used to produce several slices of 3D images which can be stacked and played back as video to monitor the physiological processes. 4D PET CT scan is the combination of two technologies, namely positron emission tomography and computer tomography, which allows the recording of dynamic movements of organs and provides accurate information on the metabolism of a tumor. Ultrasound imaging techniques are based on sound waves and are most used in gynecology for examining cornual ectopic pregnancy, whereas 4D MRI technology is a safer, radiation-free, technique that is based on radio and magnetic waves for creating images of the whole body.

The most common steps in a 4D image construction in these techniques are image acquisition, image processing, image reconstruction, and display (Kanaga et al., 2021). The material programming approach of 4D printing for wearable assistive technologies is based on biological models that adapt to environmental stimuli (Cheng et al., 2021). The 4D scaffold bioprinting process is classified into three types: (i) scaffold bio-fabrication by cell seeding and material transformation; (ii) scaffold production, by cell seeding and followed by material transformation; (iii) simultaneous scaffold production by material transformation with cell seeding (Ionov, 2018). The stimuli-responsive capabilities of bilayer polymer by using (PLA-b-PEG-b-PLA/NIPAAm) under thermo-responsive stimuli for bioabsorbable implant application that can swell and subsequently fold up under low temperatures (Pedron et al., 2011). 4D imaging in the health-care sector can revolutionize the surgical and treatment process by assisting in preoperative surgical planning by providing anatomical models replicating the natural characteristics of bone, organs, and tissue. The real process can be replicated by the use of 4D imaging to four-dimensionally print the haptic model. A 4D-capable drug delivery system can be formed with the help of details extracted from 4D imaging data of an organ and a body (Chae et al., 2015).

1.4.6 ADVANCED DRIVER-ASSISTANCE SYSTEMS

In the era of self-driving and the adoption of autonomous vehicle, 4D imaging radar can assist in safer driving and a reduced accident rate, as it utilizes a larger radio-frequency channel and signal that permits the formation of precise 4D data points per frame to provide accurate details of elevation, range, and velocity (Sun and Zhang, 2021). There are several advantages of autonomous driving, not limited to reduced traffic congestion, reduced accidents, improvement in fuel economy, and reduction in travel time. Figure 1.14 shows the bibliographic analysis for the keywords "additive manufacturing in automotive".

1.4.7 4D IMAGING IN MATERIAL MICROSCOPY

The development of 4D ultrafast electron microscopy (UFEM) permits the physicist, chemist, material scientist, and biologist to study complex phase transition, molecular reactions, and structural dynamics proceeding in femtoseconds, picoseconds, or nanoseconds in the form of video (Yang and Yasuda, 2020). By using the concept of 4D imaging, UFEM has made it possible to study highly spatial matter with high temporal resolution. 4D imaging in microscopy advances material research and is an unprecedented and revolutionary innovative technology. 4D imaging in microscopy makes it possible to analyze self-repairing ceramics processes and polymer composites, subsurface failure, the charging and discharging of fuel cells, crack growth in

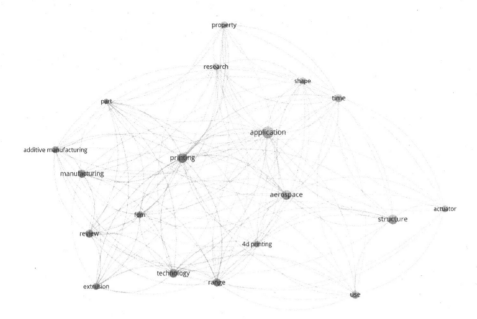

FIGURE 1.14 Bibliographic analysis for the keywords "additive manufacturing in automotive".

bioinspired structures, and hierarchal biomaterials. The behavior of smart polymeric material and smart composites can be studied using 4D imaging and, using 4D printing, functional devices for end-user applications can be fabricated. Figure 1.15 shows the bibliographic analysis for the keywords "4D printing with novel material". Based upon Figure 1.15, the research gaps have been highlighted in Figures 1.16 and 1.17 respectively.

In sensor technology, the real-time dynamic movement of a sensor can be observed using advanced 4D imaging and can be replicated by 4D printing. The development of conductive hydrogel links as a force and tactile sensor to fabricate pneumatic actuators has been outlined by Robinson et al. (2015). Smart wearables on textiles can be fabricated with the help of 4D imaging. Figure 1.18 and 1.19 respectively show bibliographic analysis for the keywords "sensor in 4D printing" and the research gap for the node as an external stimulus.

1.4.8 4D Imaging in Disaster Management

Rapid development in the meteorological sectors worldwide of earth-observation systems and geospatial technologies with 4D imaging from advanced satellites has enhanced forecasting capabilities, advance updates of weather conditions, and disaster management. The hydrometeorological data provided by multi-dimensional visualization methods and virtual reality allows analysis and monitoring of sea levels (Su et al., 2016; Li et al., 2011). 4D imaging can provide meteorologists with detailed

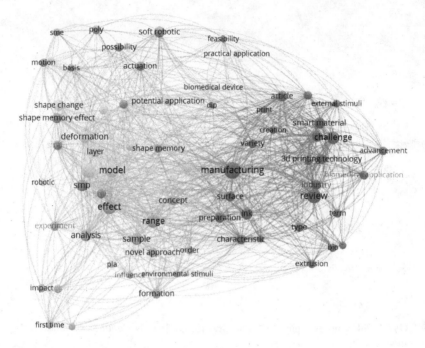

FIGURE 1.15   Bibliographic analysis for the keywords "4D printing with novel material".

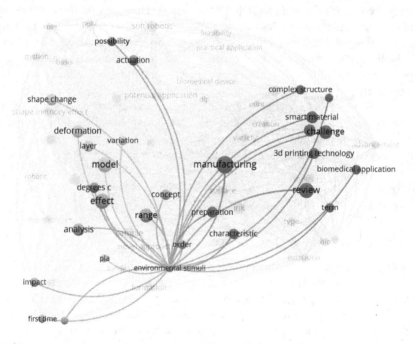

FIGURE 1.16   Research-gap analysis for "environmental stimuli".

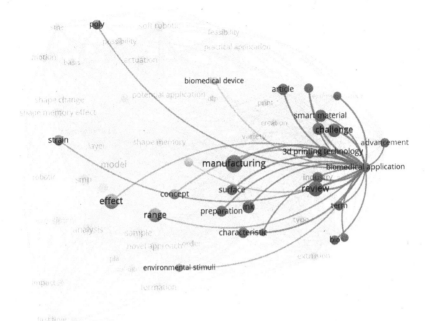

FIGURE 1.17 Research-gap analysis for "biomedical application".

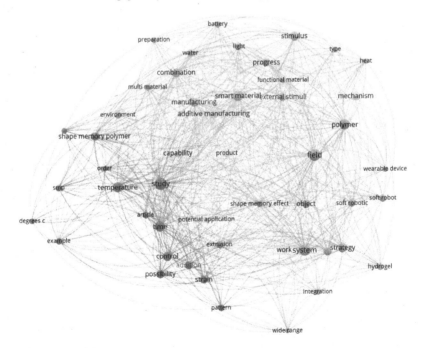

FIGURE 1.18 Bibliographic analysis for the keywords "sensor in 4D printing".

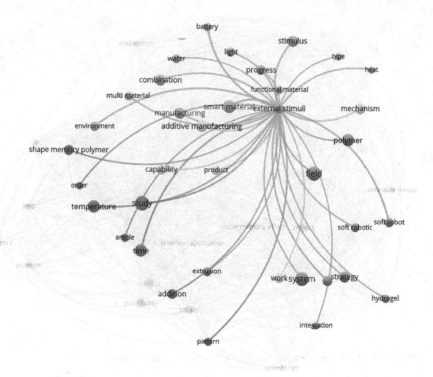

FIGURE 1.19   Research-gap analysis for "external stimuli".

information about changes in the environment, weather conditions, and emergencies, and with accurate forecasts.

1.5   CASE STUDY ON ASCERTAINING THE SURFACE PROPERTIES OF RECYCLED THERMOPLASTICS AFTER WEAR

In this case study, the surface image of abrasive wear performance was checked for acrylonitrile butadiene styrene (ABS) and Nylon 6 composite. The prepared Nylon 6 composite was fabricated using Al_2O_3 10% and Al 30% as reinforcements (Table 1.2). The wear test was performed by applying the load 20N. The surface image of ABS and Nylon 6 composite (as per Table 1.2) was captured using scanning electron microscopy (Figure 1.20 (Sample 1), Figure 1.21 (Sample 2), Figure 1.22 (Sample 3), Figure 1.23 (Sample 4)). Further, for image processing the open-source image-processing tool, Gwyddion was used to extract surface characteristics such as surface roughness (Ra), amplitude distribution function (ADF), bearing ratio curve (BRC), peak count (PC), and waviness average. It was observed from the image processing that Sample 1 underwent a wear test with a load of 20N and a sliding distance of 190m and has a surface roughness (Ra) value of 23.57nm with a waviness average of 13.28nm, whereas Sample 2 which had undergone 20N and a sliding distance of

TABLE 1.2

Compositions of Recycled Thermoplastics Prepared Composites

Sample	ABS	NYLON 6	Al	Al$_2$O$_3$
1	100	–	–	–
2	–	60	26	14
3	–	60	28	12
4	–	60	30	10

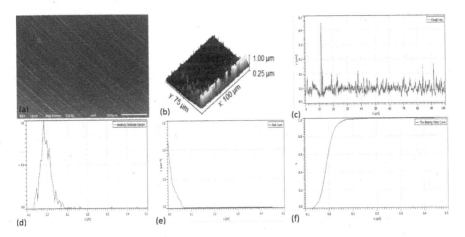

FIGURE 1.20 Sample 1 image-processing data: (a) SEM image, (b) 3D image, (c) surface roughness, (d) ADF, (e) PC, and (f) BRC.

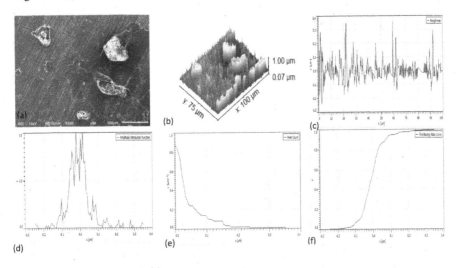

FIGURE 1.21 Sample 2 image-processing data: (a) SEM image, (b) 3D image, (c) surface roughness, (d) ADF, (e) PC, and (f) BRC.

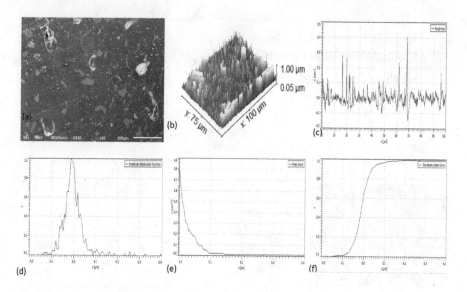

FIGURE 1.22 Sample 3 image-processing data: (a) SEM image, (b) 3D image, (c) Surface roughness, (d) ADF, (e) PC, and (f) BRC.

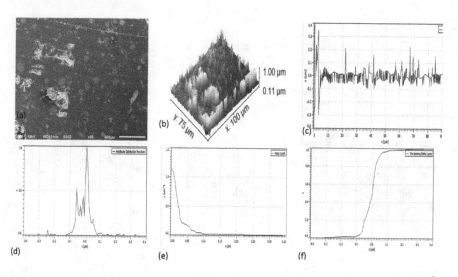

FIGURE 1.23 Sample 4 image-processing data. (a) SEM image, (b) 3D image, (c) Surface roughness, (d) ADF, (e) PC, and (f) BRC.

380m had a surface roughness (Ra) value of 49.30nm and a waviness average of 92.39nm. Similarly, in both Sample 1 and Sample 2, the ADF graph of Sample 2 has more spread, whereas Sample 1 is more uniformly distributed than Sample 2. Similarly, the bearing ratio curve of Sample 1 is flatter than Sample 2. But in the case of composites, the image processing showed opposite results for a sample processing setting load of 20N and for both Sample 3 and Sample 4 with 190 and 380 m sliding distances (m) respectively. The observed surface roughness (Ra) value of Sample 3 was 37.75 nm and a waviness average of 37.54nm and Sample 4 recorded a value of surface roughness (Ra) of 32.21nm with a waviness average of 39.09nm. The ADF has a more uniform spread in Sample 3 than in Sample 4; similarly, the bearing ratio curve of Sample 4 is flatter than in Sample 3.

1.6 SUMMARY AND OUTLOOK

The presented chapter introduces 4D imaging and its integration with 4D printing to explore new dimensions of future trends in a wide variety of applications such as health care, agriculture, quality control, Industrial Revolution 4.0, material science, food technology, drug delivery, autonomous driving, etc. Three-dimensional (3D) printing has emerged as a revolutionary manufacturing process and is essential for Industrial Revolution 4.0. In contrast to health care and biomedical applications, 3D printing fabricated parts fell short of what was expected mainly due to their inability to realistically mimic the natural conditions of soft and hard tissue. The advent of 4D printing and 4D imaging is adequately addressing the shortcomings of 3D printing and 3D imaging by incorporating the time-dependent dimension (fourth dimension) respectively. In addition to this study, the surface characteristics of recycled thermoplastics have been explored in terms of image processing to exploit their new features.

REFERENCES

Alchanatis, V., Peleg, K. and Ziv, M., 1993. Classification of tissue culture segments by colour machine vision. *Journal of Agricultural Engineering Research*, 55(4), pp. 299–311.

Carlone, L., Dong, J., Fenu, S., Rains, G. and Dellaert, F., 2015, May. Towards 4D crop analysis in precision agriculture: Estimating plant height and crown radius over time via expectation-maximization. In P. Corke and T. Drummond (Ed.), *ICRA Workshop on Robotics in Agriculture* (pp. 1–8). Australia, Brisbane: Australian Centre for Robotic Vision and Greg Hager (Johns Hopkins University).

Chae, M.P., Hunter-Smith, D.J., De-Silva, I., Tham, S., Spychal, R.T. and Rozen, W.M., 2015. Four-dimensional (4D) printing: A new evolution in computed tomography-guided stereolithographic modeling. Principles and application. *Journal of Reconstructive Microsurgery*, 31(6), pp. 458–463.

Cheng, T., Thielen, M., Poppinga, S., Tahouni, Y., Wood, D., Steinberg, T., Menges, A. and Speck, T., 2021. Bio-inspired motion mechanisms: Computational design and material programming of self-adjusting 4D-printed wearable systems. *Advanced Science*, 8(13), p. 2100411.

Dong, J., Carlone, L., Rains, G.C., Coolong, T. and Dellaert, F., 2014. 4D mapping of fields using autonomous ground and aerial vehicles. In *2014 Montreal, Quebec Canada July 13–July 16, 2014* (p. 1). St. Joseph, MI: American Society of Agricultural and Biological Engineers. www.asabe.org.

Errington, R.J., Fricker, M.D., Wood, J.L., Hall, A.C. and White, N.S., 1997. Four-dimensional imaging of living chondrocytes in cartilage using confocal microscopy: A pragmatic approach. *American Journal of Physiology-Cell Physiology*, 272(3), pp. C1040–C1051.

Grabowski, D. and Cristalli, C., 2015. Production line quality control using infrared imaging. *Infrared Physics and Technology*, 71, pp. 416–423.

Gustafson, T. and Kinnander, H., 1960. Cellular mechanisms in morphogenesis of the sea urchin gastrula: The oral contact. *Experimental Cell Research*, 21(2), pp. 361–373.

Howarth, M.S. and Searcy, S.W., 1992. Inspection of fresh carrots by machine vision. In *Food Processing Automation II: Proceedings of the 1992 Conference, 4-6 May 1992, Lexington Center* (Vol. 2950, pp. 49085–9659). Lexington, KT: Food and Process Engineering Institute.

Ionov, L., 2018. 4D biofabrication: Materials, methods, and applications. *Advanced Healthcare Materials*, 7(17), p. 1800412.

Kanaga, E.G.M., Anitha, J. and Juliet, D.S., 2021. 4D medical image analysis: A systematic study on applications, challenges, and future research directions. In T. Gandhi, S. Bhattacharyya, S. De, D. Konar and S. Dey (Ed.), *Advanced Machine Vision Paradigms for Medical Image Analysis* (pp. 97–130). Elsevier Inc.

Kriete, A. and Wagner, H.J., 1993. A method for Spatio-temporal (4-D) data representation in confocal microscopy: Application to neuroanatomical plasticity. *Journal of Microscopy*, 169(1), pp. 27–31.

Li, G., Citrin, D., Camphausen, K., Mueller, B., Burman, C., Mychalczak, B., Miller, R.W. and Song, Y., 2008. Advances in 4D medical imaging and 4D radiation therapy. *Technology in Cancer Research and Treatment*, 7(1), pp. 67–81.

Li, J. and Carayon, P., 2021. Health care 4.0: A vision for smart and connected health care. *IISE Transactions on Healthcare Systems Engineering*, 11(3), pp. 171–180.

Li, W., Chen, G., Kong, Q., Wang, Z. and Qian, C., 2011. A VR-Ocean system for interactive geospatial analysis and 4D visualization of the marine environment around Antarctica. *Computers and Geosciences*, 37(11), pp. 1743–1751.

Lin, S., Chen, J., Hertz, P. and Kahrilas, P.J., 1996. Dynamic reconstruction of the oropharyngeal swallow using computer-based animation. *Computerized Medical Imaging and Graphics*, 20(2), pp. 69–75.

Loew, L.M., Tuft, R.A., Carrington, W. and Fay, F.S., 1993. Imaging in five dimensions: Time-dependent membrane potentials in individual mitochondria. *Biophysical Journal*, 65(6), pp. 2396–2407.

Malinda, K.M., Fisher, G.W. and Ettensohn, C.A., 1995. Four-dimensional microscopic analysis of the filopodial behavior of primary mesenchyme cells during gastrulation in the sea urchin embryo. *Developmental Biology*, 172(2), pp. 552–566.

Nezhad, M.A.K.B., Massh, J. and Komleh, H.E., 2011, November. Tomato picking machine vision using with the open CV's library. In *2011 7th Iranian Conference on Machine Vision and Image Processing* (pp. 1–5). Red Hook, NY: Curran Associates, Inc.

Pedron, S., Van Lierop, S., Horstman, P., Penterman, R., Broer, D.J. and Peeters, E., 2011. Stimuli-responsive delivery vehicles for cardiac microtissue transplantation. *Advanced Functional Materials*, 21(9), pp. 1624–1630.

Raj, M.P., Swaminarayan, P.R. and Istar, A., 2015. Applications of image processing for grading agriculture products. *International Journal on Recent and Innovation Trends in Computing and Communication*, 3(3), pp. 1194–1201.

Reid, J.F. and Searcy, S.W., 1987. Automatic tractor guidance with computer vision. *SAE Transactions*, 96, pp. 673–693. https://doi.org/10.4271/871639.

Reid, J.F. and Searcy, S.W., 1991. An algorithm for computer vision sensing of a row crop guidance directrix. *SAE Transactions*, 100, pp. 93–105.

Robinson, S.S., O'Brien, K.W., Zhao, H., Peele, B.N., Larson, C.M., Mac Murray, B.C., Van Meerbeek, I.M., Dunham, S.N. and Shepherd, R.F., 2015. Integrated soft sensors and elastomeric actuators for tactile machines with kinesthetic sense. *Extreme Mechanics Letters*, 5, pp. 47–53.

Siddiqi, M.H., Ahmad, I. and Sulaiman, S.B., 2009, April. Weed recognition based on erosion and dilation segmentation algorithm. In L. O'Conner (Ed.), *2009 International Conference on Education Technology and Computer* (pp. 224–228). Los Alamitos, CA: IEEE Computer Society.

Somwang, P. and Muangklang, E., 2019, July. Image processing for quality control in manufacturing process. In *2019 16th International Conference on Electrical Engineering/ Electronics, Computer, Telecommunications and Information Technology (ECTI-CON)* (pp. 782–785). Pattaya: IEEE. http://doi.org/10.1109/ECTI-CON47248.2019 .8955421.

Su, T., Cao, Z., Lv, Z., Liu, C. and Li, X., 2016. Multi-dimensional visualization of large-scale marine hydrological environmental data. *Advances in Engineering Software*, 95, pp. 7–15.

Sun, S. and Zhang, Y.D., 2021. 4D automotive radar sensing for autonomous vehicles: A sparsity-oriented approach. *IEEE Journal of Selected Topics in Signal Processing*, 15(4), pp. 879–891.

Thomas, C.F. and White, J.G., 1998. Four-dimensional imaging: The exploration of space and time. *Trends in Biotechnology*, 16(4), pp. 175–182.

Tian, Y., Wang, L. and Zhou, Q., 2011, October. Grading method of crop disease based on image processing. In *International Conference on Computer and Computing Technologies in Agriculture* (pp. 427–433). Berlin, Heidelberg: Springer.

Turano, T.A., D'Arpa, P., Clark, W.L. and Williams, J.R., 1985. A time-lapse, image digitization video microscope system based on a mini computer with large peripheral memory. *Computers in Biology and Medicine*, 15(4), pp. 177–185.

Yang, J. and Yasuda, H., 2020. Introductory chapter: 4D imaging. In J. Yang (Ed.), *Novel Imaging and Spectroscopy*. London: IntechOpen. https://doi.org/10.5772/intechopen .92350.

2 Use of Open-Source 4D Imaging Tools for Biomedical Applications

Abhishek Kumar, Abhishek Barwar,
and Rupinder Singh

CONTENTS

2.1 INTRODUCTION

Open-source software represents different models of software evaluation or distribution for the practitioner, students, and research communities in many fields, and leads the way in terms of innovation mechanisms for the user. The success of the open-source communities-based model has built an emerging paradigm in new areas other than computer applications, such as space exploration, medical imaging, pharmaceutical development, and advanced manufacturing. Premium or, more precisely, paid-for software operates on a different model in which users without source-code access need to pay for the software license and the software companies apply conditions and restrictions. The open-source software can be shared or distributed with its source code, which allows easier availability and modification. Open-source software development projects are often led by individuals to meet their own needs or groups of individuals for users' consumption, at no cost. The open-source software development model is driven by voluntary contribution. The most common scenario in an open-source software project development is that of an individual or group writing a code to meet the need for a feature or creating entirely new software to feed a local need. Open-source development communities consist of volunteers who are highly motivated professionals and, sometimes, supremely talented programmers and developers. The motivation for voluntarily carrying out the open-source project is a combination of user need, the high reputation of high-quality open-source projects, and enjoyment in the work (Lakhani and Hippel; 2004, Caban et al., 2007; Ratib and Rosset, 2006; Wolf et al., 2005). The advantages associated with open-source software are ease of availability, ease of function, user-friendly interface, flexibility, quality, inexpensiveness, interoperability, customizability, stability, and community support. The digital transformation opportunities provided by open-source software in developing countries are worth noting. There is a significant difference between software developed by software companies and that by individuals in academic projects; the software developed by software companies is intended to fulfill market needs and to produce strong and concrete results, whereas in the academic project the developed software is for scientific novelty or it aims to serve science (Silva et al., 2017; Jodogne, 2018; Zollner et al., 2016; Caroprese et al., 2018).

To translate research outcomes from clinical trials and practice, development in biomedical informatics has pushed the boundaries to achieve professional and highly efficient and accurate clinically competent software. There is a need to identify reliable medical imaging software that can be used in clinical research for reliable results with high accuracy and repeatability. Promising biomedical software development can be completed by following the following proposed guidelines: project and team management; test-driven development with continuous feedback integration; interpretability; software distribution; a quality-driven approach; and user-centered design. Pervasive and vibrant open-source projects in biomedical informatics can lead to great inventions in the exploration of real-world health information by integrating novel modules through interdisciplinary collaboration which can accelerate the creative process. The interdisciplinary approach in medical software research can unleash creativity and integrate the knowledge from the subject domain based on the area of expertise.

2.2 MEDICAL IMAGING

Medical imaging is used as a previsualizing technique by surgeons to understand the anatomical intricacies of the subject. Medical image analysis has triggered the development of 3D, and even higher-dimensional, image datasets for treatment. Imaging software has driven the progress in biomedical and many other scientific disciplines for visualizing and analyzing volumetric biological imaging data acquired from computed tomography (CT), X-ray, and magnetic resonance imaging (MRI). Medical image processing is a subset of computer vision. In the past two decades, open-source project communities have contributed to the development of standard medical imaging visualizing and analyzing tools that can be sourced as a framework for biomedical research in computer-assisted diagnosis. It is also worth noting that there is rapid growth in interest from researchers and medical professionals to use rapid prototyping to develop new techniques, implants, and scaffolds using medical imaging data. Medical imaging data acquired during clinical trials, or for clinical purposes apart from patient diagnosis, serve legitimate secondary applications in rapid prototyping and in research libraries for deployment in multicenter trials or surgical assessment. Medical residents and surgeons exclusively rely on medical imaging data for treatment and decision-making. The development in medical imaging allows surgeons to provide targeted advanced personalized treatment to the patient. Digital imaging and communications in medicine (DICOM) are considered the gold standard for medical imaging data management in the healthcare sector; the purpose of DICOM is that of recording, capturing, and media-exchanging in picture archiving and communications systems (PACS) (Scholl et al., 2011; Yamauchi et al., 2010; Ariani et al., 2014; Ettinger et al., 2008; Haak et al., 2016).

4D imaging in healthcare has minimized the errors of 2D and 3D volumetric images caused by time and by the details of patient motion, which are inevitable but lead to uncertainty, delineation, artifact error, and localization. The 2D and 3D paradigm is advanced to 4D medical imaging which can be acquired from time-resolved computed tomography (CT), magnetic resonance imaging (MRI), and ultrasound imaging machines; these technologies utilize parallel multi-detector array for volumetric image reconstruction and accurate image projection. The advance in medical imaging has encouraged the development of digital medical image analysis software which, through open-access software's application programming interface (API), can be tailored to be patient-specific or problem-specific. The limitations of dedicated medical imaging software can be resolved by introducing modules for artifact correction, spatial image registration, quantitative feature extraction, and anatomy segmentation. The development of medical imaging software is mainly being driven by academic research communities. It is observed that open-source software development in health care is particularly focused on medical image analysis, patient medical-record management software, and picture-archiving and communication-systems (PACS) applications. Successful surgery or diagnosis of any disease relies mainly on the medical imaging data of the patient. Medical residents and surgeons need the medical imaging data in order to understand the current state of the patient, to evaluate the conditions from the empirical data or from visual judgment, and to decide on the preferred treatment (Flower, 2012) as seen in Figure 2.1.

In 1983, a joint committee made up from the National Electrical Manufacturers Association (NEMA) and the American College of Radiology (ACR) introduced the medical imaging and information standard "DICOM (.dcm file format)". The sole purpose of the DICOM standard was to facilitate PACS file use with other hospitals and medical information systems for record management and collection of medical databases which can be supplied and shared with other devices. The sharing of the medical imaging database (DICOM files) can promote faster access to medical images and faster diagnosis (C-DAC, 2015c). It accommodates most of the medical imaging formats and texture information. The development of the DICOM standard has led to greater advancement in medical imaging because of its ability to integrate with modern imaging equipment and multi-vendor equipment (Mildenberger et al., 2002). Medical imaging software is much more than an algorithm built for image visualizing; it should have the ability to process and interpret data for accurate results (Deserno, 2010). The processing of medical imaging involves five basic elements: the acquisition of the image, preprocessing of the image, image segmentation, postprocessing of the image, and image analysis. Figure 2.2 shows basic elements of medical imaging processing.

There are several medical imaging software tools available for standalone and combined features, such as DICOM viewing, DICOM preprocessing, DICOM

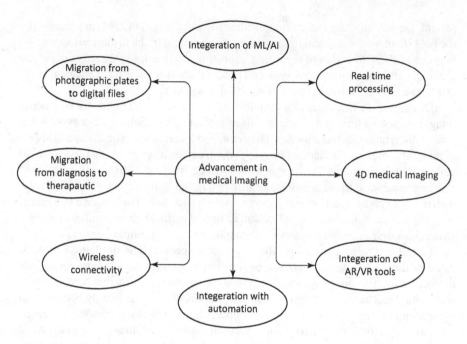

FIGURE 2.1   Advancement in medical imaging.

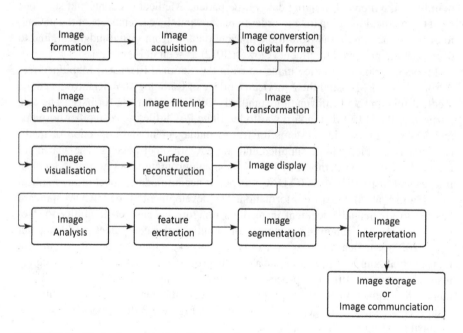

FIGURE 2.2   Basic elements of medical imaging processing.

interpretation, etc. The most commonly used DICOM software (open source and software available with the free trial for evaluation and academic purposes) are: PostDICOM (https://www.postdicom.com); RadiANT (https://www.radiantviewer .com); OsiriX Lite (https://www.osirix-viewer.com); MicroDicom (https://www.mic-rodicom.com); MANGO Multi-Image Analysis GUI (http://ric.uthscsa.edu/mango /mango.html); Escape EMV (https://escapetech.eu/index.html); Ginkgo CADx (https://ginkgo-cadx.com); Athena DICOM Viewer (https://athenadicomviewer .com); and WEASIS (https://nroduit.github.io).

To interpret and ascertain the research potential, web of science research data (database source: www.webofscience.com) has been explored for the keywords "open source 4D medical imaging" and 103 documents were discovered from the last 20 years. Further, using the open-source VOS viewer software, the research gap was analyzed in these documents and by keeping the number of keywords "3" out of 99 met the threshold. The 60% relevant keywords For the selected 99 keywords were analyzed, and the total strength of the cooccurrence link with other keywords was calculated (Table 2.1). Based on Table 2.1, Figure 2.3 shows the bibliographic analysis for the keywords "open-source 4D medical imaging"; whereas Figure 2.4 and Figure 2.5 show the bibliographic analysis for keywords "open-source software" and "X-ray imaging" respectively.

2.3 CASE STUDY ON USING OPEN-SOURCE SOFTWARE FOR VIRTUAL MODEL RECONSTRUCTION AND MAKING READY-TO-PRINT ORTHOPEDIC ANATOMY MODELS

The objective of this section is to demonstrate the use of open-source 4D imaging tools for biomedical applications. In this case study, the CT scan acquired in the DICOM file is utilized for medical imaging by the "RadiANT" DICOM viewer; open-source software (free 30 days' trial) is available on the web for educational purposes and is utilized to translate medical imaging databases for data visualization and surface reconstruction. The interpreted medical imaging data can be converted into a virtual CAD model and Standard Tessellation Language (STL format) for additive manufacturing processes.

The non-contrast computed tomography (NCCT) medical image information from cadaver specimens of the femur, tibia, and fibula bone were acquired from a CT-scan X-ray (make, Siemens SOMATOM scope observer model) with the spiral acquisition process. The obtained CT-scan X-ray was transformed to DICOM format as shown below. The CT-scan medical image shows two femur bones, tibia and fibula bone combined, and one fibula bone. Figure 2.6 shows the CT scan image of the cadaver specimens.

Further, the DICOM files were checked for 3D surface reconstruction in DICOM itself as shown in Figure 2.7.

The acquired DICOM image is then imported to RadiANT DICOM viewer software by clicking on the browser menu and selecting the open DICOM folder option. The extended feature will command prompt the file directory menu. The DICOM

TABLE 2.1
The Relevance Score for Bibliographic Analysis

S No.	Keyword	Occurrences	Relevance Score
1	Analysis	13	0.4189
2	Applicability	3	1.0958
3	Area	4	0.913
4	Capability	6	0.5157
5	Cell	7	1.1812
6	Change	6	0.5769
7	Code	3	1.9234
8	Community	4	0.8406
9	Comparison	3	1.2096
10	Contrast	8	0.6213
11	Correlation	5	0.5621
12	Dataset	6	0.8827
13	Deformation	5	0.5207
14	Depth	5	0.5342
15	Disease	5	0.5332
16	Dose	5	0.9605
17	Evolution	4	2.5303
18	Example	3	1.081
19	Experiment	10	0.4218
20	Frame	5	1.0587
21	Functionality	5	1.2371
22	Growth	4	2.215
23	Implementation	7	0.5022
24	Integration	4	0.9165
25	Limitation	3	1.6276
26	Lung	4	1.0083
27	Mechanism	5	2.4324
28	Motion	6	1.2903
29	MRI	4	1.3317
30	Number	3	1.1978
31	Oct	3	1.2158
32	Open source	6	0.5056
33	Open-source software	6	0.5491
34	Optical coherence tomography	3	1.1166
35	Orientation	3	0.9567
36	Paper	4	0.7774
37	Patient	8	0.5037
38	Performance	7	0.4552
39	Phantom	6	1.0842
40	Pipeline	6	0.7995
41	Process	10	0.8248
42	Radiotherapy	4	1.8654

(*Continued*)

TABLE 2.1 (CONTINUED)
The Relevance Score for Bibliographic Analysis

S No.	Keyword	Occurrences	Relevance Score
43	Sample	4	0.8267
44	Semantic segmentation	3	1.01
45	Simulation	8	1.0661
46	Software package	7	0.5012
47	Source code	4	0.8718
48	Stage	4	2.012
49	State	4	1.0598
50	Stem	3	0.4713
51	Surface	4	1.0643
52	Tissue	6	0.5822
53	Validation	6	0.9297
54	View	3	1.3893
55	Visualization	6	0.6471
56	Work	7	0.5567
57	Workflow	6	0.3761
58	X-ray	3	0.9562
59	X-ray imaging	4	1.0287
60	Xcat phantom	3	1.8563

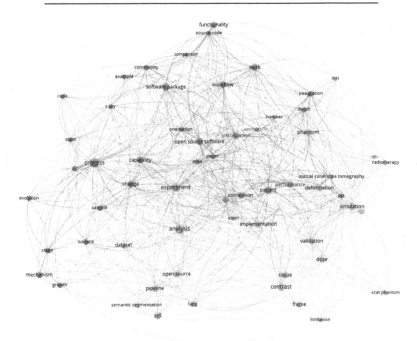

FIGURE 2.3   Bibliographic analysis for keywords "open source 4D medical imaging".

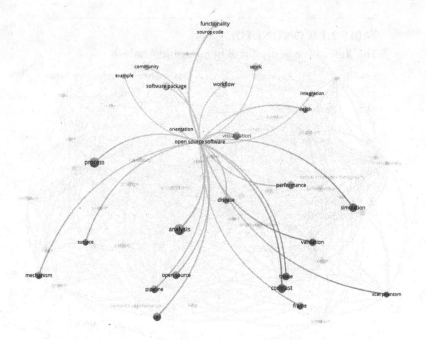

FIGURE 2.4   Bibliographic analysis for keywords "open-source software".

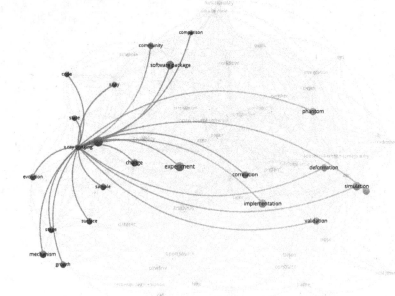

FIGURE 2.5   Bibliographic analysis for keywords "X-ray imaging".

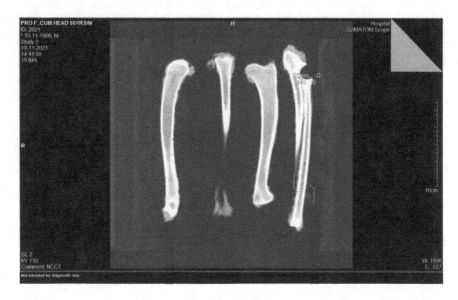

FIGURE 2.6 CT-scan image of the cadaver specimens.

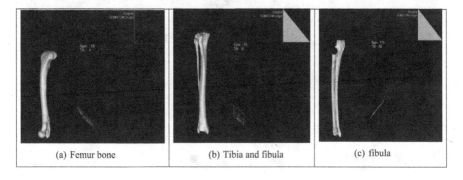

| (a) Femur bone | (b) Tibia and fibula | (c) fibula |

FIGURE 2.7 Virtual 3D surface reconstruction.

file can be selected and the import menu can be clicked on. Then, the DICOM file is imported. The imported medical image files are shown in Figure 2.8.

The top, bottom, and side views of the medical image are shown in Figure 2.9.

Surface reconstruction is carried out by adjusting the medical image in the multi-planar feature (MPR) as shown in Figure 2.10.

The virtual CAD model is developed by executing the 3D command function. The virtual CAD reconstructed model is shown in Figure 2.11. Further, the reconstructed model was checked for accuracy and exported for STL-file generation by executing the export command.

The STL-format file was further exported to 3D printing slicing software (Boparai et al., 2021; Boparai et al., 2022) for the fabrication of the femur-bone model. The

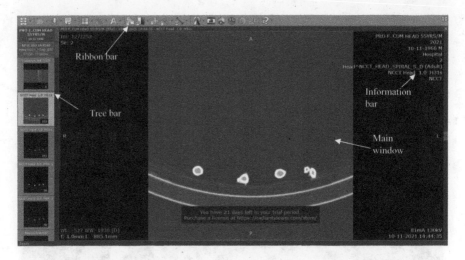

FIGURE 2.8   Imported DICOM file.

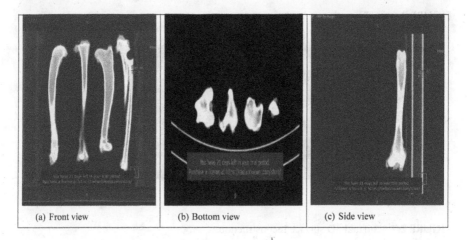

(a) Front view   (b) Bottom view   (c) Side view

FIGURE 2.9   Different orientations of the medical image.

fabricated femur-bone model may be used for preoperative surgical planning for treating the fractured femur bone. The fabricated bone model is shown in Figure 2.12. To fabricate the bone model, ABS P430 material was used on a U-print Stratasys FDM printer. The same procedure may be used for fabricating different bones.

2.4   SUMMARY AND OUTLOOK

The presented chapter highlights the use of open-source software in innovating new mechanisms for biomedical applications. In 4D medical imaging, an open-source

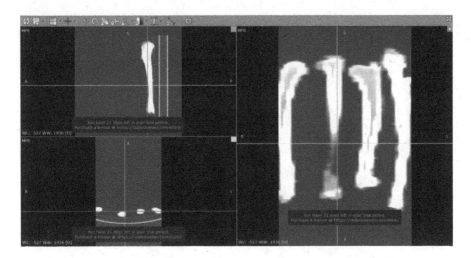

FIGURE 2.10   Multi-planar reconstruction.

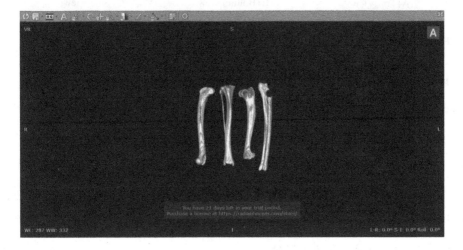

FIGURE 2.11   Virtual reconstructed models.

software model emerged as a tool for digital transformation in health care by providing users with easy availability to new features, a user-friendly interface, and integration with multiple technologies. In addition to this, the use of open-source software for fabricating ABS polymer-based bone models from DICOM data has been shown as a case study for preoperative surgical planning.

Acknowledgment: The authors are grateful to Prof. Ashwani Kumar, Veterinary Surgeon at GADVASU Ludhiana for providing DICOM data and kind guidance in supporting the case study.

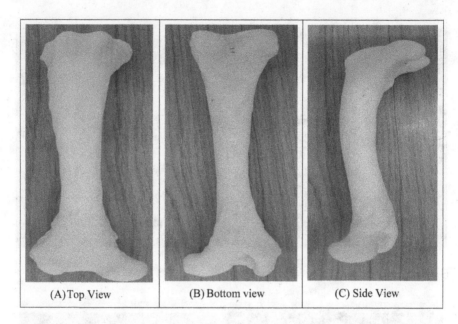

| (A) Top View | (B) Bottom view | (C) Side View |

FIGURE 2.12   3D printed femur bone.

REFERENCES

Ariani, A., Carotti, M., Gutierrez, M., Bichisecchi, E., Grassi, W., Giuseppetti, G.M. and Salaffi, F., 2014. Utility of an open-source DICOM viewer software (OsiriX) to assess pulmonary fibrosis in systemic sclerosis: Preliminary results. *Rheumatology International*, 34(4), pp. 511–516.

Boparai, K.S., Kumar, A., Kumar, A., Aman, A. and Singh, S., 2021. Nanomaterial in additive manufacturing for energy storage applications. In C.M. Hussain (Ed.), *Handbook of Polymer Nanocomposites for Industrial Applications* (pp. 529–543). Amsterdam, Netherlands: Elsevier.

Boparai, K.S., Kumar, A. and Singh, R., 2022. On characterization of rechargeable, flexible electrochemical energy storage device. In R. Singh (Ed.), *4D Printing* (pp. 67–88). Amsterdam, Netherlands: Elsevier.

Caban, J.J., Joshi, A. and Nagy, P., 2007. Rapid development of medical imaging tools with open-source libraries. *Journal of Digital Imaging*, 20(1), pp. 83–93.

Caroprese, L., Cascini, P.L., Cinaglia, P., Dattola, F., Franco, P., Iaquinta, P., Iusi, M., Tradigo, G., Veltri, P. and Zumpano, E., 2018, September. Software tools for medical imaging extended abstract. In *European Conference on Advances in Databases and Information Systems* (pp. 297–304). Cham: Springer.

C-DAC, P., Digital imaging and communications in medicine (DICOM)-PS3. 0-2015c.

Deserno, T.M., 2010. Fundamentals of biomedical image processing. In T.M. Deserno (Ed.), *Biomedical Image Processing* (pp. 1–51). Berlin, Heidelberg: Springer.

Flower, M.A. ed., 2012. *Webb's Physics of Medical Imaging*. Boca Raton, FL: CRC Press.

Haak, D., Page, C.E. and Deserno, T.M., 2016. A survey of DICOM viewer software to integrate clinical research and medical imaging. *Journal of Digital Imaging*, 29(2), pp. 206–215.

Jodogne, S., 2018. The Orthanc ecosystem for medical imaging. *Journal of Digital Imaging*, 31(3), pp. 341–352.

Lakhani, K.R. and Hippel, E.V., 2004. How open source software works: "free" user-to-user assistance. In C. Herstatt and J.G. Sander (Ed.), *Produktentwicklung mit virtuellen Communities* (pp. 303–339). Wiesbaden: Gabler Verlag Wiesbaden, Betriebswirtschaftlicher Verlag Dr. Th. Gabler/GWV Fachverlage GmbH.

Mildenberger, P., Eichelberg, M. and Martin, E., 2002. Introduction to the DICOM standard. *European Radiology*, 12(4), pp. 920–927.

Ratib, O. and Rosset, A., 2006. Open-source software in medical imaging: Development of OsiriX. *International Journal of Computer Assisted Radiology and Surgery*, 1(4), pp. 187–196.

Scholl, I., Aach, T., Deserno, T.M. and Kuhlen, T., 2011. Challenges of medical image processing. *Computer Science – Research and Development*, 26(1), pp. 5–13.

Silva, L.B., Jimenez, R.C., Blomberg, N. and Luis Oliveira, J., 2017. General guidelines for biomedical software development. *F1000Research*, 6, p. 273. https://doi.org/10.12688/f1000research.10750.2.

Van Ettinger, M.J.B., Lipton, J.A., de Wijs, M.C.J., van der Putten, N. and Nelwan, S.P., 2008, September. An open source ECG toolkit with DICOM. In A. Murray (Ed.), *2008 Computers in Cardiology* (pp. 441–444). New York: IEEE. http://www.cinc.org/.

Wolf, I., Vetter, M., Wegner, I., Böttger, T., Nolden, M., Schöbinger, M., Hastenteufel, M., Kunert, T. and Meinzer, H.P., 2005. The medical imaging interaction toolkit. *Medical Image Analysis*, 9(6), pp. 594–604.

Yamauchi, T., Yamazaki, M., Okawa, A., Furuya, T., Hayashi, K., Sakuma, T., Takahashi, H., Yanagawa, N. and Koda, M., 2010. Efficacy and reliability of highly functional open source DICOM software (OsiriX) in spine surgery. *Journal of Clinical Neuroscience*, 17(6), pp. 756–759.

Zöllner, F.G., Daab, M., Sourbron, S.P., Schad, L.R., Schoenberg, S.O. and Weisser, G., 2016. An open-source software for analysis of dynamic contrast-enhanced magnetic resonance images: UMMPerfusion revisited. *BMC Medical Imaging*, 16(1), pp. 1–13.

3 Orthopedic and Dental 4D Requirements for Veterinary Patients

Ranvijay Kumar and Rupinder Singh

CONTENTS

3.1 INTRODUCTION

3D printing nowadays is an essential manufacturing process which enables the manufacturing of functional as well as nonfunctional components in a variety of subject domains such as biomedical, aerospace, automobile, tissue engineering, sensors, medical and medicines, drug delivery, etc. 3D printing or additive manufacturing is broadly divided into processes such as material extrusion (ME), vat photo-polymerization (VP), material jetting (MJ), binder jetting (BJ), powder bed fusion (PBF), direct energy deposition (DED), and sheet lamination (SL) (Karakurt and Lin, 2020; Wang et al., 2017; Fan et al., 2020). However, with the evolution of 4D printing, the application domain is highly expanded. 4D printing is an extension of the 3D printing process, ensuring a change in the fourth dimension of time affected by external stimuli. 4D printing is crucial for biomimetic applications such as biomedical tissue engineering, sensor making, actuator design, and some robotics applications (Momenj et al., 2017; Kuang et al., 2019; Choi et al., 2015). Looking into this field, the application domain can be extended with the application of innovative materials and associated techniques. For example, polylactic acid (PLA) is one of the most used thermoplastics in biomedical applications due to its biocompatibility and non-toxicity. Along with these characteristics, PLA shows the changes in dimension under heat as a stimulus. Due to this, PLA is mostly used in 4D printing applications such as scaffolding or implants in tissue engineering for

DOI: 10.1201/9781003205531-3

veterinary patients and even the human body (Melly et al., 2020; Feng et al., 2021). Some previous researchers have reported the use of PLA as one of the shape-memory materials in different applications. Leist et al. (2017) have reported shape-memory studies on PLA for the preparation of smart textiles which are capable of changing shape on the application of external stimuli. The study investigating the shape memory of PLA has suggested that activation temperature is one of the most important parameters ensuring control of shape-memory behavior (Barletta et al., 2021). Similarly, other researchers have also reported shape-memory investigation of PLA for different applications (Zhou et al., 2015; Kuang et al., 2019; Ma et al., 2021). 3D printing and 4D printing are now commercially accepted technologies for the development of scaffolds and of implants in veterinary patients. Teixeira and Belinha (2021) have studied prosthetic limb replacement in the case of dongs. Similarly, Zhao et al. (2019) have developed the bioinspired tracheal scaffold which can act under the action of magnetic stimulus. The success and application of 3D/4D printing are largely extended by the involvement of the 4D imaging concept: 4D printing with the help of the bioimaging of human/animal organs is an example of such applications. CT and ultrasound scanning of damaged organs ensures the generation of the design files which are then treated as input in biomimetic 4D printing in tissue engineering, cell growth, and implantation applications.

Significant studies have been reported on the use of 3D printing in biomedical applications. These studies have suggested that PLA is one of the most effective materials in 4D printing as it is very sensitive to temperature stimuli. Some of the studies have reported the use of 4D printing applications, especially in veterinary patients. But, until now, little has been reported on the application of 4D imaging as the tool for 4D printing applications in veterinary patients. This study demonstrates the 4D requirement of PLA-based composites materials with the add-on of 4D imaging in the case of veterinary patients.

3.2   BACKGROUND OF THE STUDY

To check the origin and basis of the research work done in the domain of "4D printing" and "4D imaging", a database has been retrieved from the web of science source www.webofscience.com. The keywords "4D printing" and "4D imaging" have been used to search the reported research papers between the years 2000 and 2022 (see Figure 3.1). A total of 145 results have been reported for this period. Among these research papers, the greatest number of studies have been reported in the year 2021 and the statistics show that in the upcoming year the number of studies related to this topic may increase.

Among the 145 reported research papers, most studies are from the material science field (20%) and engineering (17%), followed by radiology nuclear medicine medical (13%), other science technology topics (13%), chemistry (8%), computer science (7%), instrument instrumentation (6%), physics (6%), optics (6%), and imaging science photographic technology (4%) (Figure 3.2).

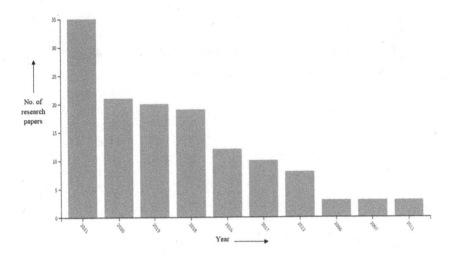

FIGURE 3.1 Year-wise publications for the domain "4D printing" and "4D imaging".

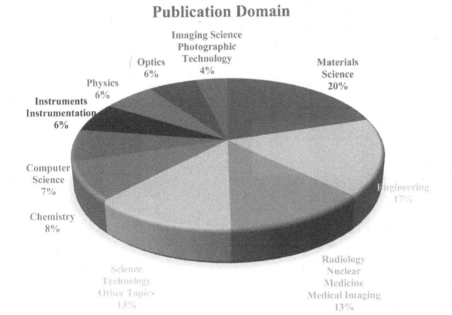

FIGURE 3.2 Publication domain for 4D printing and 4D imaging.

On analyzing the database of the 145 research papers through the bibliometric analysis software VOSviewer (version: 1.6.18), a total of 4,688 terms were found, which have been further filtered. Keeping the minimum occurrence of words in each term to 5, a total of 103 terms have been filtered and the most relevant 50 terms have been selected for the bibliometric study as given in Table 3.1.

TABLE 3.1

The Associated Term, its Occurrence, and the Relevance Score of Studies Related to 4D Printing and 4D Imaging

Sr. No.	Term	Occurrences	Relevance Score
1.	Application	45	0.6193
2.	Model	33	0.408
3.	4D printing	22	1.0188
4.	Measurement	19	0.7679
5.	Change	17	0.7054
6.	Flow	17	1.8386
7.	MRI	17	1.4026
8.	Patient	15	0.7522
9.	Response	15	0.5242
10.	Tomography	15	0.4178
11.	Architecture	14	1.1651
12.	Fabrication	14	1.1489
13.	Magnetic resonance imaging	14	1.1505
14.	Cell	13	1.2539
15.	Mechanism	13	1.1465
16.	Motion	13	0.6187
17.	Phantom	13	1.2351
18.	Geometry	12	0.1726
19.	Strategy	12	1.1973
20.	Temperature	12	0.9947
21.	Addition	11	0.4407
22.	Performance	11	0.4599
23.	Scaffold	11	1.3666
24.	Comparison	10	0.3531
25.	Evaluation	10	0.3516
26.	Formation	10	1.0572
27.	Real time	10	0.3487
28.	Construct	9	2.0268
29.	Shape-memory polymer	9	0.9944
30.	Visualization	9	0.5671
31.	Combination	8	0.6233
32.	Limitation	8	0.4506
33.	Print	8	0.6429
34.	Tissue engineering	8	1.3457
35.	Rapid prototyping	7	0.3251
36.	Algorithm	6	0.393
37.	CFD	6	2.188
38.	Hemodynamic	6	2.2112
39.	Light	6	1.5799
40.	PLA	6	0.3706

(Continued)

Sr. No.	Term	Occurrences	Relevance Score
41.	Precision	6	0.7471
42.	Smart material	6	0.9009
43.	Stereolithography	6	0.4055
44.	Vitro	6	0.9605
45.	4D flow	5	2.3568
46.	Computational fluid dynamic	5	2.1808
47.	FDM	5	0.6206
48.	Good agreement	5	1.0635
49.	Potential application	5	2.0062
50.	Validation	5	2.1238

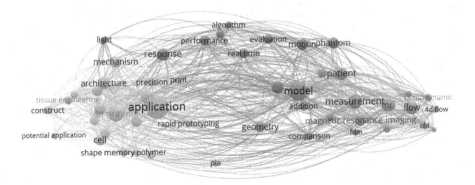

FIGURE 3.3 Bibliometric relation between the term of studies related to 4D printing and 4D imaging.

The VOSviewer software package has been used to develop the relationship diagram among the terms. It has been observed that three different clusters of the studies have been found, which are given in different clusters in Figure 3.3. It has been observed that most of the studies are related to extending the application domain by merging 4D printing and 4D imaging. Other than applications, the measurement study, model formation, architecture, precision manufacturing, real-time monitoring, response, performance, and patient-specific requirements are the major investigations of the studies. However, some gaps in the studies have been reported concerning 4D printing which may be explored in future. 4D printing studies should explore low properties, thermodynamics, and geometry so that they can best be applied, together, with 4D imaging (Figure 3.4).

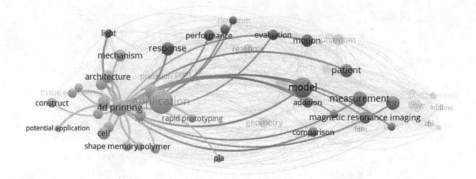

FIGURE 3.4   Gaps in the studies related to 4D printing and 4D imaging.

3.3   4D IMAGING FOR 4D PRINTING

4D imaging refers to the extension of 3D imaging in live motion and studies relating to live motion of 3D images are called 4D imaging studies. This may be understood by taking a simple example of the live body movement of the unborn baby in the mother's womb. In general terminology, this process is known as "4D ultrasound" or "4D imaging". This technique ensures better health monitoring of the baby as compared to 2D and 3D imaging. However, the better application of 4D ultrasound may be ensured by the involvement of 5D imaging which is merely the high-definition imaging of 4D ultrasound. Figure 3.5 shows the pictorial view of examples of 2D, 3D, 4D, and 5D ultrasound imaging.

In this way, the 4D imaging database may be helpful for 4D printing applications. For, example, the defective parts of the body in veterinary patients may be diagnosed with a 4D imaging tool for exact geometric monitoring and, further, 4D printing will be applied for the replacement of those defective parts by surgery.

3.4   CASE STUDY FOR THE DEVELOPMENT OF HAP-CS-BASED PLA

It has been established by the previous studies that PLA is one of the most crucial materials to be applied as scaffolds and implants in veterinary patients. Also, PLA has been declared to be a shape-memory material under the stimulus of heat/temperature. With the help of 4D imaging, the 4D printing of PLA materials may be best suited for surgical uses. Previous authors have declared that a combination of 91%PLA-8%Hap-1%CS resulted in optimum mechanical, thermal, rheological, shape-memory, and cell-culture properties (Ranjan et al., 2019; Ranjan et al., 2020). In this case study, the mechanical, thermal, rheological, and shape-memory properties reported by Ranajn et al. (2020) have been extended with process capability analysis for application in 4D printing and 4D imaging in veterinary patients. Table 3.2 shows the experimentally repeated properties of 91%PLA-8%Hap-1%CS composites. It should be noted that for five repeated experiments observations have been taken for process capability analysis.

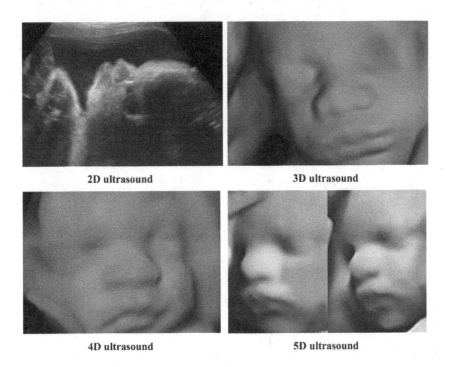

2D ultrasound   **3D ultrasound**

4D ultrasound   **5D ultrasound**

FIGURE 3.5 Example of 2D, 3D, 4D, and 5D ultrasound imaging (image courtesy: Anticipation Ultrasound studio, 2022).

TABLE 3.2
Experimental Value of Melt-Flow Index (MFI), Glass Transition Temperature (Tg), Young's Modulus, and Shape-Recovery Percentage

MFI (g/10 min)	Tg (°C)	Young's Modulus (MPa)	Shape Recovery (%)
12.35	56.50	339.22	99.82
12.86	55.21	335.58	98.56
11.84	56.04	358.82	98.85
12.04	55.86	312.84	98.45
11.86	55.89	365.85	99.05

The repeated observations of MFI, Tg, Young's modulus and shape recovery of PLA-Hap-CS composites have been drawn against the histogram plot for investigating the process capability (see Figure 3.6). It has been observed that all the experimental results are in-between the lower control limit (LCL) and the upper control limit (UCL) so that the process is statistically controlled. Similar observations have been noted in the case of normal probability plots of the MFI, Tg, Young's modulus, and shape recovery (see Figure 3.7).

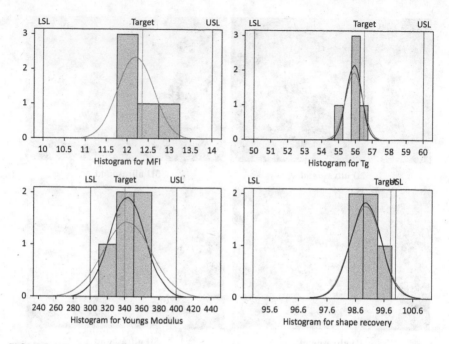

FIGURE 3.6 Histogram for MFI, Tg, Young's modulus and shape recovery of PLA-Hap-CS composites.

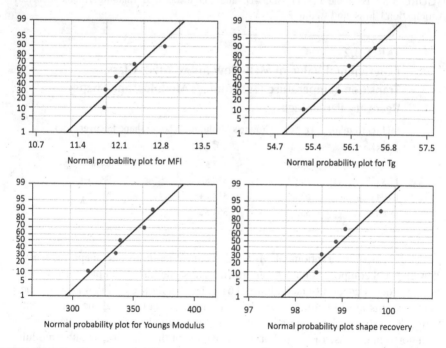

FIGURE 3.7 Normal probability plots for MFI, Tg, Young's modulus, and shape recovery of PLA-Hap-CS composites.

TABLE 3.3
Process Capability Parameters Readings for MFI of PLA-Hap-CS Composites

Readings	5	Sub-group Size	1
Tolerance Range		Data Range	
USL	14.00	Maximum	12.86
Target	12.35	Average(X-Bar)	12.1900
LSL	10.00	Minimum	11.84
Tolerance	4	Data Range	1.02
Normality Test	For AD Test: α = 0.05	Statistic	
AD Test	PASSED	Median	12.350
A-Squared	0.3641	Skewness	1.194
p Value	0.2737	Kurtosis	0.653
Potential Capability		Overall Capability	
Std. Deviation	0.423316	Std. Deviation	0.426732
Cp	1.575	Pp	1.562
Cpu	1.425	Ppu	1.414
Cpl	1.724	Ppl	1.711
Cpk	1.425	Ppk	1.414
CR	0.635	PR	0.640

The process capability analysis of the MFI of PLA-HAP-CS composite has resulted in Cp and Cpk values of 1.575 and 1.425 respectively which shows the process can give accurate outputs (see Table 3.3). Other values of the process capability analysis are in line with the values of the Cp and Cpk.

The process capability analysis of the Tg of PLA-HAP-CS composite has resulted in the Cp and Cpk values of 3.227 and 2.647 respectively which shows the process can give accurate outputs (see Table 3.4). Other values of the process capability analysis for Tg are in line with the values of the Cp and Cpk.

The process capability analysis of the Youngs modulus of PLA-HAP-CS composite has resulted in the Cp and Cpk values of 0.597 and 0.507 respectively which shows the process can give fairly accurate outputs but less so than MFI and Tg (see Table 3.5). Other values of the process capability analysis for Young's modulus are in line with the values of the Cp and Cpk.

The process capability analysis of the shape recovery of PLA-HAP-CS composite has resulted in Cp and Cpk values of 1.475 and 0.622 respectively which shows the process can give accurate outputs (see Table 3.6). Other values of the process capability analysis for shape recovery are in line with the values of the Cp and Cpk.

3.5 SUMMARY

A summary of this is as follows:

TABLE 3.4

Process Capability Parameters Readings for Tg of PLA-Hap-CS Composites

Readings	5		Sub-group Size	1
Tolerance Range			**Data Range**	
USL	60.0		Maximum	56.5
Target	56.5		Average(X-Bar)	55.9000
LSL	50.0		Minimum	55.21
Tolerance	10		Data Range	1.29
Normality Test	**For AD Test: α = 0.05**		**Statistic**	
AD Test	PASSED		Median	56.040
A-Squared	0.2877		Skewness	-0.461
p Value	0.4565		Kurtosis	1.703
Potential Capability			**Overall Capability**	
Std. Deviation	0.516401		Std. Deviation	0.462979
Cp	3.227		Pp	3.600
Cpu	2.647		Ppu	2.952
Cpl	3.808		Ppl	4.248
Cpk	2.647		Ppk	2.952

TABLE 3.5

Process Capability Parameters Readings for Young's Modulus of PLA-Hap-CS Composites

Readings	5		Sub-group Size	1
Tolerance Range			**Data Range**	
USL	400.00		Maximum	365.85
Target	339.22		Average(X-Bar)	342.4620
LSL	300.00		Minimum	312.84
Tolerance	100		Data Range	53.01
Normality Test	**For AD Test: α = 0.05**		**Statistic**	
AD Test	PASSED		Median	358.820
A-Squared	0.2206		Skewness	-0.418
p Value	0.6660		Kurtosis	-0.534
Potential Capability			**Overall Capability**	
Std. Deviation	27.896720		Std. Deviation	20.916011
Cp	0.597		Pp	0.797
Cpu	0.688		Ppu	0.917
Cpl	0.507		Ppl	0.677
Cpk	0.507		Ppk	0.677
CR	1.674		PR	1.255

TABLE 3.6

Process Capability Parameters Readings for Shape Recovery of PLA-Hap-CS Composites

Readings	5	Sub-group Size	1
Tolerance Range		**Data Range**	
USL	100.00	Maximum	99.82
Target	99.82	Average(X-Bar)	98.9460
LSL	95.00	Minimum	98.45
Tolerance	5	Data Range	1.37
Normality Test	**For AD Test: α = 0.05**	**Statistic**	
AD Test	PASSED	Median	99.050
A-Squared	0.3197	Skewness	1.272
p Value	0.3696	Kurtosis	1.590
Potential Capability		**Overall Capability**	
Std. Deviation	0.565160	Std. Deviation	0.542890
Cp	1.475	Pp	1.535
Cpu	0.622	Ppu	0.647
Cpl	2.327	Ppl	2.423
Cpk	0.622	Ppk	0.647
CR	0.678	PR	0.651

- The success and application of 3D/4D printing are largely extended by the involvement of the 4D imaging concept. 4D printing, with the help of the bioimaging of human/animal organs, is an example of such applications.
- 4D printing studies should be explored with low properties, thermodynamics, and geometry so that they can best be applied together with 4D imaging.
- The defective parts of the body of veterinary patients may be diagnosed with the 4D imaging tool for exact geometric monitoring and, further, 4D printing will be applied for the replacement of those defective parts by surgery.
- The results of process capability analysis have shown that the MFI, Tg, Young's modulus and shape recovery of the PLA-HAP-CS are statistically controlled in repeating experimentation.

3.6 ACKNOWLEDGMENT

The authors are very grateful to the Science and Engineering Research Board (SERB) (File Number: TAR/2021/000126) and the University Center for Research and Development, Chandigarh University for financial/technical assistance.

REFERENCES

Anticipation Ultrasound Studio. https://anticipationultrasoundstudio.com/the-difference -between-2d-3d-4d-and-5d-ultrasounds/. Retrieved on 01 June 2022.

Barletta, M., Gisario, A. and Mehrpouya, M., 2021. 4D printing of shape memory polylactic acid (PLA) components: Investigating the role of the operational parameters in fused deposition modeling (FDM). *Journal of Manufacturing Processes*, 61, pp. 473–480.

Choi, J., Kwon, O.C., Jo, W., Lee, H.J. and Moon, M.W., 2015. 4D printing technology: A review. *3D Printing and Additive Manufacturing*, 2(4), pp. 159–167.

Fan, D., Li, Y., Wang, X., Zhu, T., Wang, Q., Cai, H., Li, W., Tian, Y. and Liu, Z., 2020. Progressive 3D printing technology and its application in medical materials. *Frontiers in Pharmacology*, 11, p. 122.

Feng, P., Jia, J., Liu, M., Peng, S., Zhao, Z. and Shuai, C., 2021. Degradation mechanisms and acceleration strategies of poly (lactic acid) scaffold for bone regeneration. *Materials and Design*, 210, p. 110066.

Karakurt, I. and Lin, L., 2020. 3D printing technologies: Techniques, materials, and post-processing. *Current Opinion in Chemical Engineering*, 28, pp. 134–143.

Kuang, X., Roach, D.J., Wu, J., Hamel, C.M., Ding, Z., Wang, T., Dunn, M.L. and Qi, H.J., 2019. Advances in 4D printing: Materials and applications. *Advanced Functional Materials*, 29(2), p. 1805290.

Leist, S.K., Gao, D., Chiou, R. and Zhou, J., 2017. Investigating the shape memory properties of 4D printed polylactic acid (PLA) and the concept of 4D printing onto nylon fabrics for the creation of smart textiles. *Virtual and Physical Prototyping*, 12(4), pp. 290–300.

Ma, S., Jiang, Z., Wang, M., Zhang, L., Liang, Y., Zhang, Z., Ren, L. and Ren, L., 2021. 4D printing of PLA/PCL shape memory composites with controllable sequential deformation. *Bio-Design and Manufacturing*, 4(4), pp. 867–878.

Melly, S.K., Liu, L., Liu, Y. and Leng, J., 2020. On 4D printing as a revolutionary fabrication technique for smart structures. *Smart Materials and Structures*, 29(8), p. 083001.

Momeni, F., Liu, X. and Ni, J., 2017. A review of 4D printing. *Materials and Design*, 122, pp. 42–79.

Ranjan, N., Singh, R. and Ahuja, I.P., 2020. Development of PLA-HAp-CS-based bio-compatible functional prototype: A case study. *Journal of Thermoplastic Composite Materials*, 33(3), pp. 305–323.

Ranjan, N., Singh, R., Ahuja, I.P. and Singh, J., 2019. Fabrication of PLA-HAp-CS based biocompatible and biodegradable feedstock filament using twin-screw extrusion. In Dr. B. AlMangour (Ed.), *Additive Manufacturing of Emerging Materials* (pp. 325–345). Cham: Springer.

Teixeira, M. and Belinha, J., 2021. Prosthetic limb replacement in dogs. In J. Belinha, J.C.R. Campos, E. Fonseca, M.H.F. Silva, M.A. Marques, M.F.G. Costa and S. Oliveira (Eds.), *Advances and Current Trends in Biomechanics* (pp. 438–441). Boca Raton, FL: CRC Press.

Wang, X., Jiang, M., Zhou, Z., Gou, J. and Hui, D., 2017. 3D printing of polymer matrix composites: A review and perspective. *Composites Part B: Engineering*, 110, pp. 442–458.

Zhao, W., Zhang, F., Leng, J. and Liu, Y., 2019. Personalized 4D printing of bioinspired tracheal scaffold concept based on magnetic stimulated shape memory composites. *Composites Science and Technology*, 184, p. 107866.

Zhou, Y., Huang, W.M., Kang, S.F., Wu, X.L., Lu, H.B., Fu, J. and Cui, H., 2015. From 3D to 4D printing: Approaches and typical applications. *Journal of Mechanical Science and Technology*, 29(10), pp. 4281–4288.

4 A Case Study for Dentistry Application Using Medical Imaging

Abhishek Kumar, Smruti Ranjan Pradhan,
Rupinder Singh, and Vaibhav Sahani

CONTENTS

4.1 INTRODUCTION

In clinical dentistry, the classical workflow which was once considered standard practice – such as acquiring alginate impressions for primary cast fabrication in prosthodontics, relying on 2D and 3D imaging for treating dentomaxillofacial structures, designing gypsum-based dental templates for orthodontics – is constantly being replaced by more advanced digital approaches which are considered more efficient and accurate (Rekow, 2020; Joda et al., 2020). Earlier treatment modalities involved the fabrication of radiographic templates that the patient wore for the radiographic acquisition. These radiographic templates had radio-opaque markers which would then be converted to a surgical template. With the advent of digital workflow in dental implantology, all that is required is the patient DICOM file along with the STL data. This not only simplifies the process of surgical template fabrication but also enhances communication between members of the dental team as well as with the patient (Flugge et al., 2017; Lanis and Del canto, 2015). Digitalization in clinical dentistry includes computer-assisted surgical guidance tools and covers broader areas such as patient data acquisition and collection using high-end image modalities, application of computer-aided design and computer-aided manufacturing (CAD/CAM) resources, treatment planning, patient assessment, clinical diagnosis, etc. (Lin, 2018). The advances in CAD/CAM aid dental clinicians in performing dentomaxillofacial treatment with virtual planning and treatment using 3D printing (Shujaat et al., 2021).

Endosseous implants have made possible the rehabilitation of completely and partially edentulous individuals (Adell et al., 1981, 1990; Branemark et al., 1977;

Botticelli et al., 2005). Traditionally, implant placement protocols have involved placement in healed extraction sites. In the late 1980s, evidence began to emerge of implants being placed immediately post-exodontia (Lazzara,1989). To supplement these procedures, augmentation was performed by the utilization of barrier membranes to preserve the ridge anatomy and cut down on overall treatment times (Becker et al., 1994a, 1994b; Becker and Sennerby, 1999). The reliability of immediately placed dental implants has been confirmed in numerous studies (Grunder et al., 1999; Schwartz and Chashu, 1997a; Wagenberg and Froum, 2006; Schwartz and Chashu, 1997b). A variety of grafting materials have been utilized to fill the gap between the implant and the adjacent bone to improve clinical outcomes. Autografts, allografts, xenografts as well as alloplasts have all been utilized to provide improved clinical outcomes, particularly in the immediate implant placement setting (Mellonig and Nevins, 1995; Hermann and Buser, 1996; Nevins and Jovanovic, 1997). The stability of implants so placed has been amenable to verification via a variety of methodologies, with the most non-invasive of these perhaps being resonance frequency analysis (RFA) (Meredith, 1997a, 1997b).

RFA involves the utilization of a transducer on the abutment or head of the implant itself which is then subjected to a current of low voltage (~ 1V). These currents are of no consequence to the patient. The current, by virtue of its passage through a transducer, gives rise to vibrations, the transducer-level resistance to which is registered digitally.

Initially, RFA values were recorded in Hertz. This was later adapted into what is termed the implant stability quotient (ISQ) (Petersson and Sennerby, 2016).

$$ISQ = \frac{\left(Measured\ Frequency - min.frequency\right)}{\left(max.frequency - min.frequency\right)} \times 100$$

It is generally accepted that implants demonstrating ISQ values north of 50 would be stable clinically. Primary stability values tend to be lower for the maxilla as compared to the mandible. This may be due to the greater cancellous to cortical bone ratio in the maxilla as compared to the mandible. This can be attributed, among other factors, to the quality of bone. These values tend to achieve equitability by the end of the first year as healing ensues.

Exodontia may be indicated for a variety of reasons, some of which may include insufficient tooth dimensions and crown: root proportions, non-restorable fractures of the teeth, and root resorption.

In the so-called "aesthetic zone", the contour of the periodontium, bone levels, gingival display upon smiling, and the morphology of the former need to be evaluated before treatment is initiated (Ochsenbein and Ross, 1969).

Inter-implant distance, as well as the availability of bone in the periphery of the proposed implant sites, along with the adjacent contact relations, need to be accounted for (Becker et al., 1997).

In certain situations, wherein the soft tissue is deemed to be inadequate, adjunctive or interdisciplinary procedures such as those involving orthodontic extrusion before extraction may be necessitated. As the tooth is forcefully extruded, the bone and gingival levels tend to move coronally as well, essentially augmenting the future implant site with natural tissue. Soft tissue deficiencies may also be addressed by the grafting procedures where indicated (Tarnow et al., 1992, 2003; Langer and Langer, 1990).

Radiography involves an evaluation of not only the quantity but also the quality and morphology of the site in question. Additionally, it aids in the demarcation of vital structures such as nerves, vasculature, and sinuses, which need to be respected before the implant is placed (Worthington, 2004).

If extraction has to be undertaken, the reasons for this should be justifiable. This does not imply heroic attempts to save seemingly hopeless dentition. The growing body of literature on the success and predictability of dental implants has caused a paradigm shift in treatment planning. It is now regarded as an act of prudence to be able to identify dentition that would fail to remain amenable for a variety of reasons and to remove appropriate teeth to be rehabilitated with dental implants. Virtual planning plays a major role in determining eventual clinical outcomes by enhancing the predictability of the procedure at various levels. The digital planning workflow for dental implants requires radiographic data in three dimensions (DICOM) along with data derived from scanning casts or the oral cavity of the patient. The latter is available in STL format. The generation of a surgical template involves importing both the DICOM and STL data sets into a planning software which essentially superimposes these by the utilization of certain registration or matching points. These points are generally maintained on hard tissue. Such a process aids in the alignment of the data sets to provide for a more meaningful outcome. Any doubts as to the accuracy of the superimposition must be addressed to arrive at the most suitable fit as an improperly fabricated surgical guide is problematic during the surgical procedure. Additionally, improperly placed implants can have severe consequences for the patient. Another important aspect involves marking vital structures, such as the inferior alveolar nerve, on the planning software. Being the most frequently traumatized nerve during oral surgery, a distance of at least 1.5 mm must be maintained between the implant and the nerve (Tay and Zuniga, 2007). The identification of morphological features, such as undercuts in the bone, can also aid in avoiding iatrogenic errors such as those of perforating bony plates during the drilling sequence. Implant planning software already contains data about different implant types. Alternatively, such designs may be imported into the software from an external source. The planning stage also allows for ascertaining the angulation and exact positioning of the future osteotomy site and, by that extension, the implant itself. In cases where the surgeon has not performed the planning steps himself or herself, these must be validated thoroughly before proceeding with the surgery (Sammartino et al., 2008; Vercruyssen et al., 2015).

Computer-guided implant surgery, on the other hand, involves the incorporation of fiducial markers in radiographic templates, which essentially act as a representative for the planned prosthetic aspect of the treatment plan. Radiography, generally a cone-beam computed tomography (CBCT) scan, is then performed, with the patient wearing said appliance. The DICOM data so obtained can then be imported into implant planning software or standalone image manipulation software. Current generation implant planning software, such as coDiagnostiX, NobelClinician, and VIPSoftware, facilitate the transfer of the proposed treatment plant directly to a CAD/CAM center which would, in turn, design and manufacture the surgical guides/templates. The manufacturing processes involved can be computerized drilling or stereolithography/additive manufacturing. Traditional impression techniques have involved the utilization of a variety of impression materials, such as alginate and addition silicones, to obtain impressions to pour casts; these are utilized at various stages of the diagnosis and treatment planning process. While these methods continue to be utilized, the advent of digital impression techniques appears to provide a viable alternative to the more traditional methods of impression making. Digital impression techniques obviate the need for the presence of impression materials inside the oral cavity and thus tend to facilitate patient acceptability. These also eliminate the otherwise remote possibility of an allergic reaction to these materials. Digital impression techniques involve the acquisition and transfer of scan data for cast fabrication. Current generation modalities also facilitate the fabrication of diagnostic casts with implant analogs, further enhancing the utility of this technology (Schwarz et al., 1987a, 1987b).

The web of science (WOS) research database global collection has been scanned by putting in the keywords "4D imaging in dentistry" to identify the research gap. The research database literature collection (2006–2022) has shown a total of 48 publications on the topic of 4D imaging in dentistry. The bibliometric analysis was performed using the open-source freeware VOSviewer by analyzing the keywords provided by the authors. The minimum occurrences of keywords were set to 3 of the 1,896 terms out of which 86 terms met the threshold limit. From the selected 86 terms, a relevance score of 60% for the most relevant term has been calculated as a "52" term. Figure 4.1

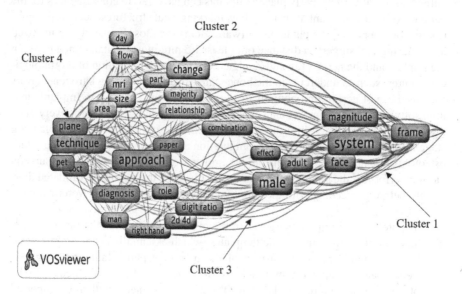

FIGURE 4.1   The bibliographic analysis of the keywords "4D imaging in dentistry".

shows the bibliographic analysis of the keywords "4D imaging in dentistry". In bibliometric analysis, 4 clusters have been formed for the 52 relevant terms. The formed cluster was analyzed for understanding the closeness of relevant terms with nodes (Tables 4.1–4.4).

TABLE 4.1
Cluster 1 for the Bibliographic Analysis of the Keywords "4D Imaging in Dentistry"

S. No	Keyword	Occurrences	Relevance Score
1	4D Imaging	3	0.9435
2	Cheek Puff	3	0.9331
3	Dynamic	4	0.8146
4	Face	5	0.6803
5	Facial Asymmetry	3	0.9245
6	Facial Landmark	3	0.6098
7	Frame	5	0.9568
8	Landmark	7	0.551
9	Lip Purse	3	0.9331
10	Magnitude	4	0.6578
11	Maximal Smile	3	0.7946
12	Maximum Smile	3	1.2942
13	Reproducibility	3	1.6021
14	Rest	4	0.828
15	System	11	0.5585

TABLE 4.2
Cluster 2 for the Bibliographic Analysis of the Keywords "4D Imaging in Dentistry"

S. No	Keyword	Occurrences	Relevance Score
1	Area	7	1.0147
2	Change	7	0.5964
3	day	4	2.1035
4	flow	3	1.7259
5	hemodynamic	3	1.8715
6	literature	3	0.9732
7	Majority	4	0.6513
8	mechanism	5	1.2817
9	MRI	6	0.8772
10	Part	3	0.8416
11	relationship	3	0.5694
12	size	5	0.9898
13	stage	3	1.6392

TABLE 4.3

Cluster 3 for the Bibliographic Analysis of the Keywords "4D Imaging in Dentistry"

S. No	Keyword	Occurrences	Relevance score
1	2D 4D	4	1.3385
2	Adult	5	0.6598
3	Combination	4	0.8031
4	Digit ratio	4	1.3109
5	Effect	3	0.9374
6	Gene	3	1.6276
7	Male	10	0.4546
8	Man	3	1.4217
9	Radiation therapy	3	1.1225
10	Right hand	3	1.4912
11	Role	5	0.8244
12	Woman	3	1.4217

TABLE 4.4

Cluster 4 for the Bibliographic Analysis of the Keywords "4D Imaging in Dentistry"

S. No	Keyword	Occurrences	Relevance Score
1	3D reconstruction	3	1.2101
2	Approach	10	0.3513
3	CBCT	3	1.0698
4	Cone beam	4	1.0289
5	diagnosis	4	0.5922
6	Image fusion	3	1.2128
7	paper	3	0.304
8	Pet	3	1.2149
9	Plane	5	1.1053
10	point	5	0.52
11	Process	7	0.9448
12	technique	9	0.8154

4.2   METHODOLOGY FOR TOOTH DATA EXTRACTION FROM MEDICAL IMAGING SOFTWARE

Digitization of the implant diagnostic and therapeutic workflow has distinct advantages over more traditional methods. While the latter still maintain their usefulness in many respects, the digital component seems to provide increasingly more viable and acceptable alternatives while altogether replacing conventional methodologies in certain situations. Once the exact positioning of the implant has been fixed, this is then transferred into the design process for the surgical template. A partial, or fully, guided approach may be utilized at this stage. The partially guided approach only provides a guide for the initial pilot drill. A fully guided approach involves supplementing the surgical guide with multiple sleeves to guide each sequential drill. Upon completion of the design stage, the template is exported as an STL file which is then subjected to CAD/CAM procedures that can be either additive or subtractive.

The manufactured surgical template is then checked for its fit inside the oral cavity at the time of the implant surgery. Such checks must be confirmed before the actual surgical procedure is commenced. Traditional methods involve raising a mucoperiosteal flap after a crestal or sub-crestal incision. The edentulous site is then subjected to a sequential drilling protocol to prepare the osteotomy site to receive the selected implant. It is at this stage that the utilization of precisely fabricated surgical templates can aid in enhancing outcomes.

Upon accomplishing the preparation of the osteotomy site, the implant is then inserted at a set torque.

The digital workflow in tooth data extraction using medical imaging in all dental specialties mostly shares a common point for virtual planning, dental restoration, implant placement, treatment planning, and surgical assessment (Lamoral et al., 1990). The common methodology used for the tooth data extraction for additive manufacturing is shown in Figure 4.2.

The transformation of medical imaging from 2D and 3D to 4D medical imaging has advanced dental treatment procedures by providing dental surgeons with more accurate patient data. The 4D medical imaging system has eliminated the drawbacks of conventional medical imaging procedures because it is capable of capturing the patient's jaw motion. Radiographs also aid in ascertaining the proper angulation of the adjacent dentition which eventually determines the parallelism which would

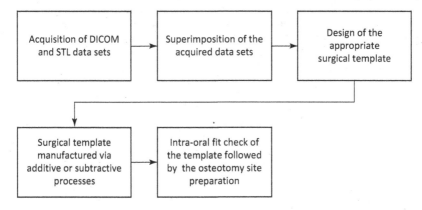

FIGURE 4.2 Workflow depicting the transition from and incorporation of virtual implant planning to the surgical setting.

need to exist between the implant to be placed. The advent of image manipulation software such as Materialise Mimics (Materialise NV, Belgium) has made possible the manipulation of DICOM data obtained from sources such as computed tomography. These images can then be reconstructed to provide a three-dimensional render of the field of interest. Such data can be utilized for the design and fabrication of surgical guides which are useful in ensuring the proper location and angulation of osteotomies during the implant placement procedure. Further, the availability of a three-dimensional view of the field can aid the clinician in visualizing and augmenting diagnostic knowledge of the region to be operated upon. These steps tend to enhance clinical outcomes.

The incorporation of 4D medical imaging in dental prosthetics has integrated patient-specific real-time motion in CAD which can provide more detailed information on the patient's case. In addition to this, 4D medical imaging system can generate detailed high-resolution six-degrees-of-freedom 3D surface data. The diagnosis and treatment planning steps for dental implant placement are followed by the actual surgical procedure to accomplish what has been planned. The placement of dental implants with adequate diameter and length into appropriate edentulous sites involves a specifically detailed surgical procedure. The incorporation of a virtual planning component carries several obvious advantages over the more traditional methods. While conventional protocols have their place, an additional virtual component enhances the entire workflow to increase predictability and eventual clinically successful outcomes. Radiographic data which is amenable to digital manipulation can aid in visualizing root angulations, distance from vital structures, and the quality and quantity of bone. This data, in conjunction with that of the surface anatomy (derived using scanning casts or intra-oral scans), can then provide a more holistic view of the oral cavity, which allows for template fabrication and guided surgery.

The workflow of tooth data extraction using medical imaging software consists of data acquisition of the subject site in the first step using image modalities such as CT-scanner and X-ray machine setups. Clinically, it is vital to have a precise and accurate imaging chain for the creation of sufficient data for the subject assessment. In addition to this, the collected data should also be sufficient for the reconstruction of a 3D surface anatomical model.

Image segmentation is the most critical, and the second, step in generating the virtual 3D anatomical model of the desired region. The unwanted captured region might be removed and the desired region can be extracted from the collected data for virtual CAD model reconstruction. Figure 4.3 shows the collected DICOM data of the tooth for translation into a virtual model. The virtual model is ready for export to STL format for additive manufacturing purposes.

The human tooth data is further processed for extracting detailed information about surface characteristics and features such as surface roughness (Ra), 3D rendered image, amplitude distribution frequency (ADF), bearing ratio curve (BRC), and peak count (PC). The surface roughness plot depicts the change in dimensional features along the different axes of rotation.

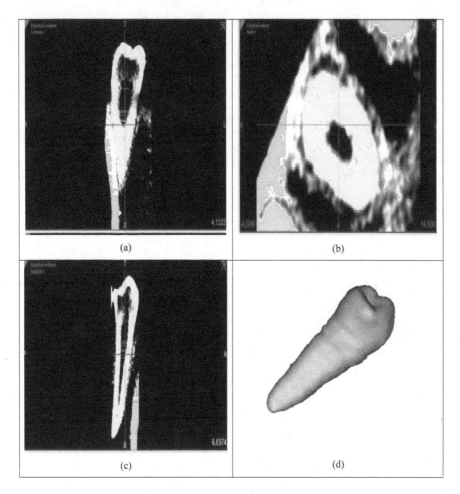

FIGURE 4.3 Translation of DICOM data to virtual model for a single tooth utilizing Materialise Mimics (Materialise NV, Belgium).

Implant surgery may now be conducted in a computer-guided fashion. This involves the utilization of a surgical template derived from DICOM data using CAD/CAM technology. Surgical templates based on the traditional cast methodologies do not simultaneously account for the multitude of prosthetic and anatomic factors which need to be thought about while considering the use of such a device to accomplish implant surgery. The result is a guide that fails to provide three-dimensional guidance with an acceptable level of accuracy (Figure 4.4).

Nowadays, additive manufacturing technology is rapidly evolving from a prototype fabrication process to a product fabrication process in multidisciplines (Boparai et al., 2021a, 2021b, 2022a, 2022b, 2016). It enables the user to fabricate and tailor products according to need and to their wishes; in addition, additive manufacturing

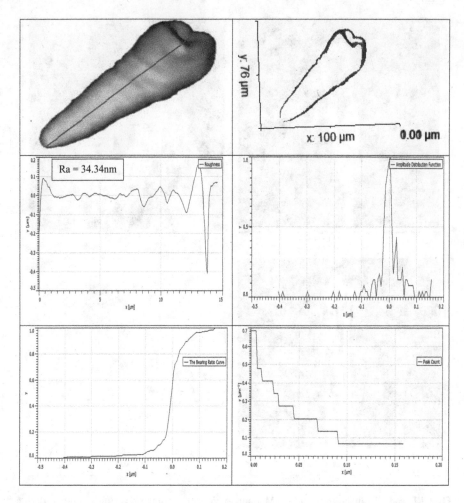

FIGURE 4.4 Surface texture analysis of the human tooth. (a) 3D rendered image; (b) 2D scanned surface; (c) Surface roughness (Ra) profile; (d) Amplitude distribution function (ADF); (e) Bearing ratio curve (BRC); (f) Peak count (PC).

provides users with easy-to-use accessibility, reduction in machine setup cost, labor cost, etc. (Singh et al., 2018a, 2018b; Pradhan et al., 2021a; Chohan et al., 2020, 2016,). Canine species used for military and surveillance purposes are more prone to dental damage and trauma; the advent of additive manufacturing can assist the surgeon with virtual surgical planning, dental treatment, and surgery of canine patients (Pradhan et al., 2021b, 2021c).

The similar case for canine teeth being three-dimensionally printed with the FDM process has been explored by using image processing; the corresponding surface characteristic features have been explored, such as surface roughness (Ra), three-dimensionally rendered image, amplitude distribution frequency (ADF), bearing ratio curve (BRC), peak count (PC). The surface roughness plot depicts the change in dimensional features along the different axes of rotation (Figure 4.5).

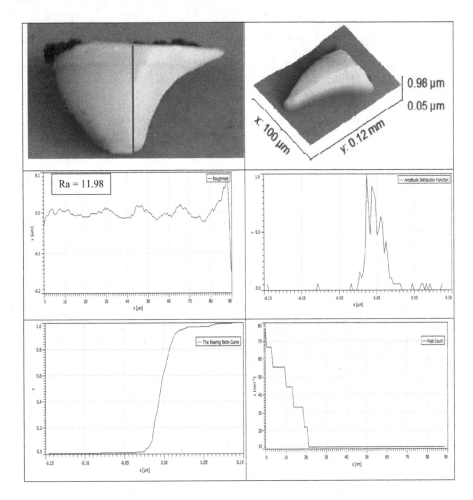

FIGURE 4.5 Surface texture analysis of canine tooth.

4.3 SUMMARY AND FUTURE OUTLOOK

Medical imaging provides the clinical dentist with a digital workflow to accumulate the data for preoperative assessment, planning, and subject-site monitoring for postoperative follow-up. Therefore, the 4D imaging data provides essential information required for treating the subject site and eliminating the error of 2D and 3D imaging data. The shortcomings of 2D and 3D imaging data significantly influences the clinical efficiency and efficacy of the digital workflow.

REFERENCES

Adell, R., Eriksson, B., Lekholm, U., Brånemark, P.I. and Jemt, T., 1990. A long-term follow-up study of osseointegrated implants in the treatment of totally edentulous jaws. *International Journal of Oral & Maxillofacial Implants*, 5(4), pp. 347–359.

Adell, R., Lekholm, U., Rockler, B. and Brånemark, P.I., 1981. A 15-year study of osseointe-grated implants in the treatment of the edentulous jaw. *International Journal of Oral Surgery*, 10(6), pp. 387–416.

Becker, W., Dahlin, C., Becker, B.E., Lekholm, U., Van Steenberghe, D., Higuchi, K. and Kultje, C., 1994a. The use of e-PTFE barrier membranes for bone promotion around titanium implants placed into extraction sockets: A prospective multicenter study. *International Journal of Oral & Maxillofacial Implants*, 9(1), pp. 31–40.

Becker, W., Becker, B.E., Polizzi, G. and Bergstrom, C., 1994b. Autogenous bone grafting of bone defects adjacent to implants placed into immediate extraction sockets in patients: A prospective study. *International Journal of Oral & Maxillofacial Implants*, 9(4), pp. 389–396.

Becker, W., Ochsenbein, C., Tibbetts, L. and Becker, B.E., 1997. Alveolar bone anatomic profiles as measured from dry skulls: Clinical ramifications. *Journal of Clinical Periodontology*, 24(10), pp. 727–731.

Becker, W. and Sennerby, L., 1999. A new era. *Clinical Implant Dentistry & Related Research*, 1(1), pp. 1.

Boparai, K.S., Singh, R. and Singh, H., 2016. Development of rapid tooling using fused deposition modeling: A review. *Rapid Prototyping Journal*, 22(2), pp. 281–299.

Boparai, K.S., Kumar, A., Kumar, A., Aman, A. and Singh, S., 2021a. Nanomaterial in additive manufacturing for energy storage applications. In C.M. Hussain (Ed.), *Handbook of Polymer Nanocomposites for Industrial Applications* (pp. 529–543). Amsterdam, Netherlands: Elsevier.

Boparai, K.S. and Kumara, A., 2021b. *Thermosetting Polymers as Scaffold Applications*. Amsterdam, Netherlands: Elsevier.

Boparai, K.S., Kumar, A. and Singh, R., 2022a. On characterization of rechargeable, flexible electrochemical energy storage device. In R. Singh (Ed.), *4D Printing* (pp. 67–88). Amsterdam, Netherlands: Elsevier.

Boparai, K.S., Kumar, A. and Singh, R., 2022b. Primary and secondary melt processing for plastics. In R. Singh and R. Kumar (Eds.), *Additive Manufacturing for Plastic Recycling* (pp. 51–65). Boca Raton, FL: CRC Press.

Botticelli, D., Berglundh, T., Persson, L.G. and Lindhe, J., 2005. Bone regeneration at implants with turned or rough surfaces in self-contained defects: An experimental study in the dog. *Journal of Clinical Periodontology*, 32(5), pp. 448–455.

Branemark, P.I., Hansson, B.O., Adell, R., Breine, U., Lindström, J., Hallén, O. and Ohman, A., 1977. Osseointegrated implants in the treatment of the edentulous jaw. Experience from a 10-year period. *Scandinavian Journal of Plastic & Reconstructive Surgery Supplementum*, 16, pp. 1–132.

Chohan, J.S., Singh, R. and Boparai, K.S., 2016. Parametric optimization of fused deposition modeling and vapour smoothing processes for surface finishing of biomedical implant replicas. *Measurement*, 94, pp. 602–613.

Chohan, J.S., Singh, R. and Boparai, K.S., 2020. Vapor smoothing process for surface finishing of FDM replicas. *Materials Today: Proceedings*, 26, pp. 173–179.

Flügge, T., Derksen, W., Te Poel, J., Hassan, B., Nelson, K. and Wismeijer, D., 2017. Registration of cone beam computed tomography data and intraoral surface scans–A prerequisite for guided implant surgery with CAD/CAM drilling guides. *Clinical Oral Implants Research*, 28(9), pp. 1113–1118.

Grunder, U., Polizzi, G., Goené, R., Hatano, N., Henry, P., Jackson, W.J., Kawamura, K., Köhler, S., Renouard, F., Rosenberg, R., Triplett, G., Werbitt, M. and Lithner, B., 1999. A 3-year prospective multicenter follow-up report on the immediate and delayed-immediate placement of implants. *International Journal of Oral & Maxillofacial Implants*, 14(2), pp. 210–216.

Hermann, J.S. and Buser, D., 1996. Guided bone regeneration for dental implants. *Current Opinion in Periodontology*, 3, pp. 168–177.

Joda, T., Bornstein, M.M., Jung, R.E., Ferrari, M., Waltimo, T. and Zitzmann, N.U., 2020. Recent trends and future direction of dental research in the digital era. *International Journal of Environmental Research & Public Health*, 17(6), pp. 1987.

Lamoral, Y., Quirynen, M., Peene, P., Vanneste, P., Lemahieu, S.P., Baert, A.L. and van Steenberghe, D., 1990, November. Computed tomography in the preoperative planning of oral endo-osseous implant surgery. In *RöFo-Fortschritte auf dem Gebiet der Röntgenstrahlen und der bildgebenden Verfahren* (Vol. 153, No. 11, pp. 505–509). New York: © Georg Thieme Verlag Stuttgart. https://doi.org/10.1055/s-2008-1033428.

Langer, B. and Langer, L., 1990. Overlapped flap: A surgical modification for implant fixture installation. *The International Journal of Periodontics & Restorative Dentistry*, 10(3), pp. 208–215.

Lanis, A. and Del Canto, O.Á., 2015. The combination of digital surface scanners and cone beam computed tomography technology for guided implant surgery using 3Shape implant studio software: A case history report. *International Journal of Prosthodontics*, 28(2), pp. 169–178.

Lazzara, R.J., 1989. Immediate implant placement into extraction sites: Surgical and restorative advantages. *International Journal of Periodontics & Restorative Dentistry*, 9(5), pp. 332–343.

Lin, Y.M., 2018. Digitalisation in dentistry: Development and practices. In Y.-C. Kim and P.-C. Chen (Eds.), *The Digitization of Business in China* (pp. 199–217). Cham: Palgrave Macmillan.

Mellonig, J.T. and Nevins, M., 1995. Guided bone regeneration of bone defects associated with implants: An evidence-based outcome assessment. *International Journal of Periodontics & Restorative Dentistry*, 15(2), pp. 168–185.

Meredith, N., Books, K., Fribergs, B., Jemt, T. and Sennerby, L., 1997b. Resonance frequency measurements of implant stability in viva: A cross-sectional and longitudinal study of resonance frequency measurements on implants in the edentulous and partially dentate maxilla. *Clinical Oral Implants Research*, 8(3), pp. 226–233.

Meredith, N., Shagaldi, F., Alleyne, D., Sennerby, L. and Cawley, P., 1997a. The application of resonance frequency measurements to study the stability of titanium implants during healing in the rabbit tibia. *Clinical Oral Implants Research*, 8(3), pp. 234–243.

Nevins, M. and Jovanovic, S.A., 1997. Localized bone reconstruction as an adjunct to dental implant placement. *Current Opinion in Periodontology*, 4, pp. 109–118.

Ochsenbein, C. and Ross, S., 1969. A reevaluation of osseous surgery. *Dental Clinics of North America*, 13(1), pp. 87–102.

Petersson, A., Ph, E. and Sennerby, L., 2016. On standard calibration of ISQ transducer pegs. *Prerequisites for Accurate and Comparable RFA Measurements. Integr Diagnostics Updat*, 1, pp. 1–3.

Pradhan, S.R., Singh, R., Banwait, S.S., Singh, S. and Anand, A., 2021a. *3D Printing Assisted Dental Crowns for Veterinary Patients* (Vol. 1, pp. 1–7). Amsterdam, Netherlands: Elsevier Inc.

Pradhan, S.R., Singh, R. and Banwait, S.S., 2021b. On crown fabrication in prosthetic dentistry of veterinary patients: A review. *Advances in Materials & Processing Technologies*, pp. 1–20. https://doi.org/10.1080/2374068X.2021.1970991.

Pradhan, S.R., Singh, R., Banwait, S.S., Puhal, M.S., Singh, S. and Anand, A., 2021c. A comparative study on investment casting of dental crowns for veterinary dentistry by using ABS patterns with and without wax coating. In R. Bennacer (Ed.), *E3S Web of Conferences (Vol. 309)*. Les Ulis Cedex A: EDP Sciences.

Rekow, E.D., 2020. Digital dentistry: The new state of the art—Is it disruptive or destructive? *Dental Materials*, 36(1), pp. 9–24.

Sammartino, G., Marenzi, G., Citarella, R., Ciccarelli, R. and Wang, H.L., 2008. Analysis of the occlusal stress transmitted to the inferior alveolar nerve by an osseointegrated threaded fixture. *Journal of Periodontology*, 79(9), pp. 1735–1744.

Schwartz-Arad, D. and Chaushu, G., 1997a. Placement of implants into fresh extraction sites: 4 to 7 years retrospective evaluation of 95 immediate implants. *Journal of Periodontology*, 68(11), pp. 1110–1116.

Schwartz-Arad, D. and Chaushu, G., 1997b. The ways and wherefores of immediate placement of implants into fresh extraction sites: A literature review. *Journal of Periodontology*, 68(10), pp. 915–923.

Schwarz, M.S., Rothman, S.L., Rhodes, M.L. and Chafetz, N., 1987a. Computed tomography: Part I. Preoperative assessment of the mandible for endosseous implant surgery. *International Journal of Oral & Maxillofacial Implants*, 2(3), pp. 137–141.

Schwarz, M.S., Rothman, S.L., Rhodes, M.L. and Chafetz, N., 1987b. Computed tomography: Part II. Preoperative assessment of the maxilla for endosseous implant surgery. *International Journal of Oral & Maxillofacial Implants*, 2(3), pp. 143–148.

Shujaat, S., Bornstein, M.M., Price, J.B. and Jacobs, R., 2021. Integration of imaging modalities in digital dental workflows-possibilities, limitations, and potential future developments. *Dento Maxillo Facial Radiology*, 50(7), p. 20210268.

Singh, D., Singh, R. and Boparai, K.S., 2018a. Development and surface improvement of FDM pattern based investment casting of biomedical implants: A state of art review. *Journal of Manufacturing Processes*, 31, pp. 80–95.

Singh, D., Singh, R., Boparai, K.S., Farina, I., Feo, L. and Verma, A.K., 2018b. In-vitro studies of SS 316 L biomedical implants prepared by FDM, vapor smoothing and investment casting. *Composites Part B: Engineering*, 132, pp. 107–114.

Tarnow, D., Elian, N., Fletcher, P., Froum, S., Magner, A., Cho, S.C., Salama, M., Salama, H. and Garber, D.A., 2003. Vertical distance from the crest of bone to the height of the interproximal papilla between adjacent implants. *Journal of Periodontology*, 74(12), pp. 1785–1788.

Tarnow, D.P., Magner, A.W. and Fletcher, P., 1992. The effect of the distance from the contact point to the crest of bone on the presence or absence of the interproximal dental papilla. *Journal of Periodontology*, 63(12), pp. 995–996.

Tay, A.B.G. and Zuniga, J.R., 2007. Clinical characteristics of trigeminal nerve injury referrals to a university centre. *International Journal of Oral & Maxillofacial Surgery*, 36(10), pp. 922–927.

Vercruyssen, M., Laleman, I., Jacobs, R. and Quirynen, M., 2015. Computer-supported implant planning and guided surgery: A narrative review. *Clinical Oral Implants Research*, 26, pp. 69–76.

Wagenberg, B. and Froum, S.J., 2006. A retrospective study of 1,925 consecutively placed immediate implants from 1988 to 2004. *International Journal of Oral & Maxillofacial Implants*, 21(1), pp. 71–80.

Worthington, P., 2004. Injury to the inferior alveolar nerve during implant placement: A formula for protection of the patient and clinician. *International Journal of Oral & Maxillofacial Implants*, 19(5), pp. 731–734.

5 Low-Cost, Indigenous, Lab-Scale Solutions for Various Biomedical Applications of Veterinary Patients: Clinical Dentistry and Orthopedics

Anish Das, Abhishek Kumar, and Rupinder Singh

CONTENTS

5.1 INTRODUCTION

The use of 3D printing in health care provides numerous advantages such as the fabrication of tailored/customized medical implants for dental and orthopedic applications using patient-specific medical imaging data. The medical imaging data for acquisition is captured usually by magnetic resonance imaging (MRI), computed

DOI: 10.1201/9781003205531-5

tomography (CT) scan, and ultrasonography. The flexibility of additive manufacturing (AM) processes to fabricate patient-specific medical implants makes it more suitable than other traditional manufacturing practices. The medical imaging data captured by different medical modalities are saved usually in DICOM format. The virtual model is further reconstructed by image segmentation to convert into a standard triangulate language (STL) extension, which is used for 3D printing. The fracture of long bones is most common in canine patients due to trauma, sudden impact, aging, and vehicle accidents. The use of rigid fixation is standard in fracture fixation to restore bone function. The rigid fixation is carried out by exposing the skin.

The workflow in AM integrated with 3D printing in orthopedics and dentistry for virtual surgical planning, implant fabrication, and functional prototypes is presented in this chapter. AM in medical applications is not restricted to the fabrication of anatomical models but includes the fabrication of bone substitutes for replacing defected areas, improving the strength of implants, producing lightweight medical implants to overcome stress shielding, and aesthetic and reconstructive surgery.

In the medical industry, AM has been deployed as a cost-effective and adaptable approach for fabricating geometrically complicated products (Li et al., 2020). It is a collection of production methods used to turn a three-dimensional (3D) digital model into a three-dimensional (3D) physical item through layer-by-layer material depositions (Sames et al., 2016). AM has also been used to create personalized medical equipment, allowing finished goods to be tailored to the patient's specific needs while being produced at relatively low cost (Novakov et al., 2017). Personalized implants and prostheses have become the gold-standard approach in recent years and are a trusted solution for patients who require particular structures (Gebhardt et al., 2010). Nowadays, dental items, such as dental implants and crowns, are commonly manufactured using additive manufacturing. AM techniques have been applied in various areas for biomedical applications. In this chapter, we focus on the development of AM for the fabrication of dental implants that are used on a particular lab scale at the clinical level. The use of biomaterials in processes such as 3D printing to develop functional prototypes for 3D application areas, including clinical dentistry and veterinary sciences has proven that novel, cost-effective, and highly customized 3D solutions may be offered for the benefit of present and future generations (Singh et al., 2017).

To ascertain the research gap, a detailed bibliographic analysis has been performed based on the database extracted from the "web of science" platform for the past 20 years. The keywords "multi-rooted teeth" and "4D imaging" were searched combinedly on the web of science database platform and the refined (web of science indexed) literature was obtained for the research that has occurred in the past two decades. The research data from the existing literature was obtained in the form of a plain text file, and is imported into the VOSviewer software (bibliographic analysis tool). At the beginning of the analysis, the minimum number of occurrences of a term was selected as 3, based upon the total of 4,121 terms extracted from the literature. Out of these terms, 273 meet the threshold value, and based upon this, the networking diagram (Figure 5.1) has been constructed which contains five clusters that represent the major research reported in a particular area of application.

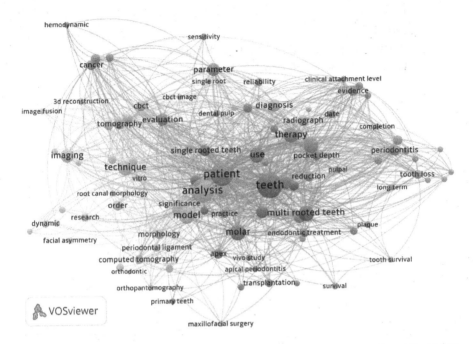

FIGURE 5.1 Bibliographic diagram based on the keywords "multi-rooted teeth" and "4D imaging".

Table 5.1 contains the information of the terms extracted from the literature obtained through the web of science database. The number of occurrences of a term and, based on that, the relevance score for a particular term was calculated in the VOSviewer software itself. Based on the relevance score of the terms, 60% of the most relevant terms contribute to the construction of a bibliographic diagram.

Further, to perform the gap analysis, the node's multi-rooted teeth and 4D imaging have been highlighted in Figure 5.2 and Figure 5.3 from the main networking diagram (Figure 5.1) respectively.

5.2 METHODOLOGY

The fabrication of low-cost dental implants as biomedical applications for veterinary patients in clinical dentistry is the subject of this case study. Design and fabrication of multi-root dental implants (MRDIs) for canines using 4D imaging and 3D printing with biocompatible material as a smart rapid tool may be regarded as novel work in the area of biomedical AM.

5.2.1 STEP 1: SELECTION OF FRACTURE TOOTH

Tooth fractures account for a significant portion of all dental problems. Because they are predominantly a result of activity in everyday life, fractures in strategic teeth

TABLE 5.1
Relevance Score and Number of Occurrences of the Terms Used to Draw the Network Diagrams

Id	Term	Occurrences	Relevance Score
1	3D Reconstruction	4	1.5176
2	4D Imaging	3	6.3717
3	Active Periodontal Therapy	3	1.2719
4	Analysis	46	0.0806
5	Apex	8	1.0405
6	Apical Periodontitis	3	0.8997
7	Benefit	7	0.5577
8	Canal	6	0.4527
9	Cancer	9	1.0662
10	Cbct	9	1.0657
11	Cbct Image	3	1.7776
12	Clinical Attachment Level	3	1.4257
13	Completion	3	0.9113
14	Computed Tomography	7	1.0794
15	Cone Beam	9	1.1444
16	Crown	7	0.899
17	Date	6	0.9078
18	Dental Pulp	4	0.6581
19	Dentistry	5	1.6835
20	Diagnosis	13	0.1894
21	Dynamic	5	4.5674
22	Effect	12	0.3752
23	Effectiveness	5	0.5478
24	Electronic Apex Locator	4	1.8793
25	Endodontic Treatment	6	0.5719
26	Evaluation	12	0.307
27	Evidence	8	1.0084
28	Extraction	14	0.2642
29	Facial Asymmetry	3	3.8773
30	Feasibility	4	1.3544
31	Furcation Involvement	8	0.7058
32	Gingival Recession	3	0.5036
33	Hemodynamic	3	2.7376
34	Image Fusion	3	1.7248
35	Imaging	16	1.2607
36	Long Term	3	0.8267
37	Magnetic Resonance Imaging	6	1.3982
38	Magnitude	4	3.4443
39	Maxillofacial Surgery	3	1.4706
40	Mechanism	8	1.1024
41	Medline	4	1.4164

(*Continued*)

Id	Term	Occurrences	Relevance Score
42	Meta Analysis	5	1.4715
43	Model	23	0.1893
44	Molar	20	0.307
45	Morphology	8	0.9209
46	MRI	8	1.2643
47	Multi-Rooted Teeth	20	0.1774
48	Non-surgical Periodontal Treatment	3	1.2691
49	Order	9	0.4468
50	Orthodontic	3	1.8628
51	Orthopantomography	3	1.4695
52	Parameter	14	0.3928
53	Patient	46	0.0991
54	Periapical Radiolucency	3	0.5753
55	Periodontal Disease	4	0.9985
56	Periodontal Ligament	6	0.9248
57	Periodontal Patient	3	1.4816
58	Periodontitis	11	0.7369
59	Periodontitis Patient	5	0.527
60	Plaque	4	0.6637
61	Pocket Depth	7	0.6486
62	Practice	7	0.4083
63	Primary Teeth	3	1.2327
64	Probability	4	1.0178
65	Procedure	21	0.2341
66	Progression	4	0.4476
67	Pulpal	3	0.7016
68	Radiograph	10	0.2926
69	Reconstruction	3	1.1561
70	Reduction	8	0.2521
71	Reliability	5	0.27
72	Reproducibility	4	1.9128
73	Research	6	2.0563
74	Retrospective Study	4	0.5593
75	Root Canal	10	0.6115
76	Root Canal Morphology	3	1.6375
77	Root Canal Treatment	8	0.4275
78	Root Length	3	0.7536
79	Sensitivity	4	0.6863
80	Significance	8	0.3654
81	Single Root	3	0.9971
82	Single-rooted Teeth	11	0.2738
83	Soft Tissue	7	0.5558
84	Specimen	6	0.7284
85	Statistical Analysis	5	0.9749
86	Supportive Periodontal Therapy	3	1.5338
87	Surgery	10	0.5207

(Continued)

TABLE 5.1 (CONTINUED)
Relevance Score and Number of Occurrences of the Terms
Used to Draw the Network Diagrams

Id	Term	Occurrences	Relevance Score
88	Survival	4	0.5283
89	Technique	18	0.4034
90	Teeth	54	0.0782
91	Therapy	19	0.2247
92	Tomography	11	1.0621
93	Tooth Extraction	5	0.6599
94	Tooth Loss	7	0.893
95	Tooth Survival	3	0.9259
96	Transplantation	5	0.5407
97	Treatment	19	0.1597
98	Type	12	0.1818
99	Use	19	0.2821
100	Vitro	4	1.0371
101	Vivo Study	3	0.644

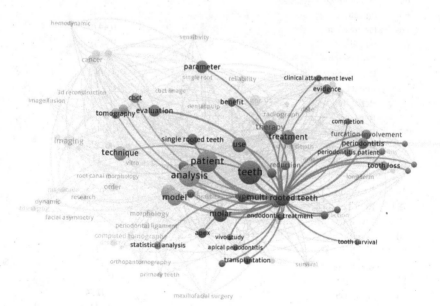

FIGURE 5.2 Research gap analysis by highlighting the nodes "multi-rooted teeth".

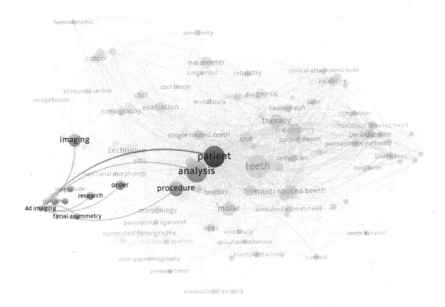

FIGURE 5.3 Research gap analysis by highlighting the nodes "4D imaging".

(ST) are highly prevalent (38.8% canine, 25.9% incisors, 2.2% molar, and 33.1% premolar) (Pradhan et al., 2021). Any partial or complete loss of the ST renders these animals ineffective, and patients cease eating. Finally, some patients may die as a result of this (Box et al., 2018). The right maxillary 4th premolar (PM4) ST, of a three-year-old male German Shepherd, shown in Figure 5.4, was undertaken for this case study.

5.2.2 STEP 2: 3D SCANNING

The extracted (from a cadaver) PM4 tooth was brought into the clinical laboratory for 3D scanning using the 3Shape E3 dental lab scanner (Figure 5.5).

5.2.3 STEP 3: STANDARD TRIANGULATION LANGUAGE (STL) FILE GENERATION

3D-Sprint, unique software for preparing and optimizing CAD data, was used in this study.

5.2.4 STEP 4: MEASUREMENT OF DIMENSIONS

Different dimensions have been acquired for implant design using SOLIDWORKS measurement tools, bearing in mind that the root makes up two-thirds of the overall length and the crown makes up the remaining one-third from the apex as shown in Figure 5.6 (Coffman et al., 2019).

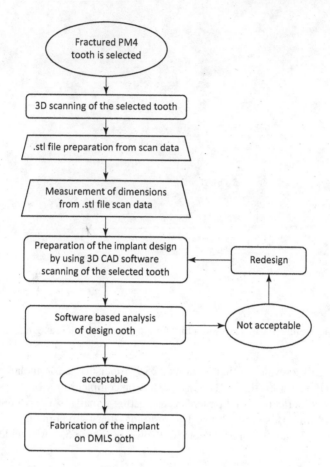

FIGURE 5.4   Adopted methodology for this study.

5.2.5   STEP 5: IMPLANT DESIGN

Implant design aims to replicate all three natural roots seen in the premolar (PM4) canine tooth. Primary stability, secondary stability, and screw-loosening issues were all taken into consideration while developing the implant, as they are the most prevalent reasons for implant failure. The MRDI assembly in Figure 5.7a consists of eight parts. The implant's apical one-third component for the longest root, the proximal root, is built as a threaded cylinder, as illustrated in Figure 5.7b, for secure and excellent anchoring, which will offer primary stability. The 3D-printed apical one-third was fixed with an appropriate armamentarium using the guiding pin in Figure 5.7c. For greater secondary stability, the middle region, i.e., the cervical part of an implant, has high porosity as illustrated in Figure 5.7d. The threaded and porous sections of the proximal root implant were aligned using a guide pin (Figure 5.7c) with one side threaded. The guide portion is positioned

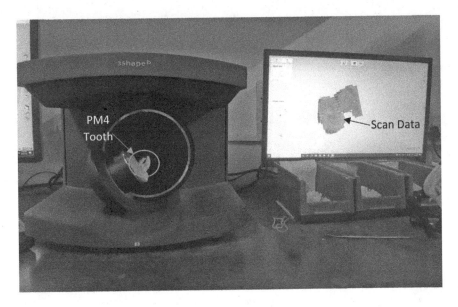

FIGURE 5.5 3Shape E3 dental lab scanner scanning PM4 tooth along with 3D-Sprint Basic for handling scan data.

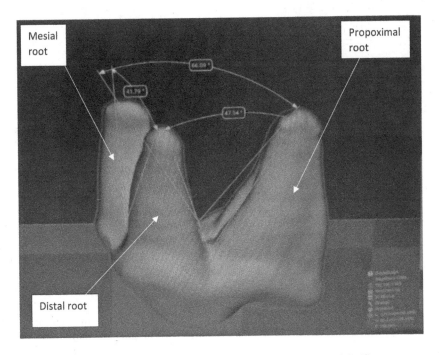

FIGURE 5.6 Measurement of dimension on the STL file in SOLIDWORKS.

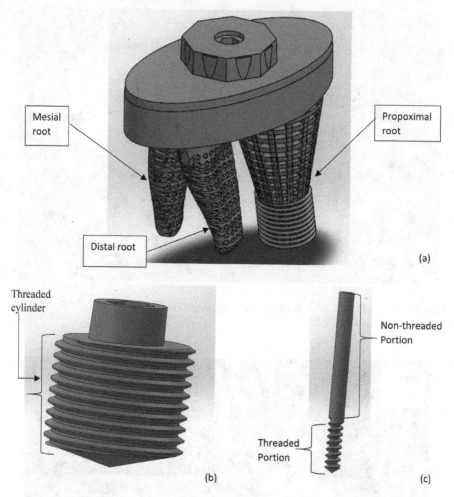

FIGURE 5.7 3D model of MRDI assembly parts designed in SOLIDWORKS.

over the cervical component and is aligned through the guide pin. The remaining two roots – mesial, the smallest root (Figure 5.7g), and distal, the medium-sized root (Figure 5.7h) – were designed with their natural complicated shapes in mind for secondary stability. From the bottom to the top the apical and middle portions were designed to be porous and the cervical part was solid with Morse taper. A fixture was designed as shown in Figure 5.7i with an equivalent thickness of the cervical height of the crown of the PM4 tooth, i.e., 0.7 mm, to hold these three components of the implant, i.e., the propoximal, mesial, and distal of the implant. Finally, a screw (Figure 5.7j) was used to secure the assembly, which will prevent horizontal displacement in the event of shear stress. SOLIDWORKS was used to develop all of the CAD files.

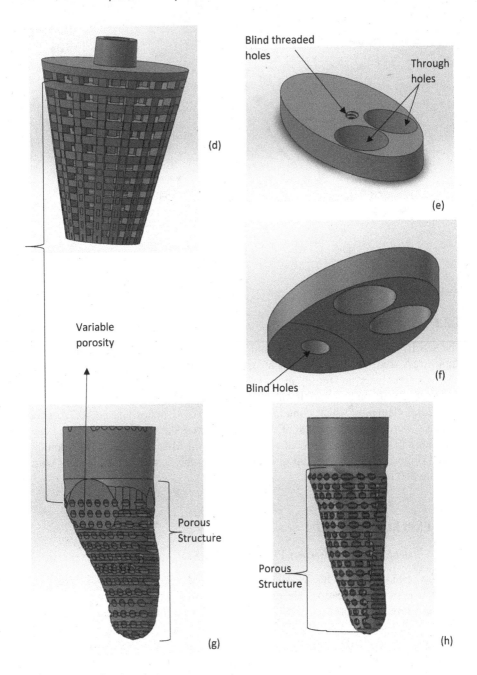

FIGURE 5.7 Continued

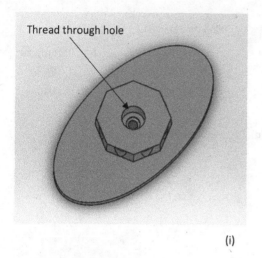

Thread through hole

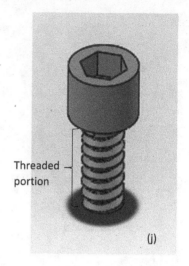

Threaded portion

(i)

(j)

FIGURE 5.7   Continued

5.2.6   STEP 6: ANALYSIS

The SOLIDWORKS simulation program was used to perform a finite element-based static-stress study. For simulations of osseointegrated implant pieces, the implant parts were combined and represented as a unit with its abutment, At the bone-implant contact, a "fixed bond" situation was established. The blended curvature-based solid tetrahedral elements, which contain roughly 24,70,477 nodes and 16,40,276 solid elements, were used to mesh the 3D model. The stress distributions were calculated using an 850 N static axial occlusal load. The Von Mises stress analysis demonstrated (Figure 5.8) that the proposed implant assembly is safe and capable of withstanding 850 N force.

5.3   EXPERIMENTATION

5.3.1   FABRICATION OF IMPLANT PARTS ON DMLS

Because of biocompatibility, 17-4 precipitation hardened (PH) stainless steel (SS) was chosen for the fabrication. The material was heated at 80°C for 24 hours to eliminate moisture. The Solidworks-2021 CAD files for MRDI components were converted to STL files and transferred into 3D System's 3DXpert software. Following that, the orientation, support type, and support height were all modified, and a fab file with auto-placement mode across the build plate with a volume of 140 × 140 × 100 mm³ was developed for full-scale printing. The fab file is then exported to the ProX® DMP200 system. N₂ gas was utilized to generate an inert environment in the machine chamber. Post-heat treatment was performed to eliminate residual stress and enhance mechanical characteristics. Implant pieces and support structures

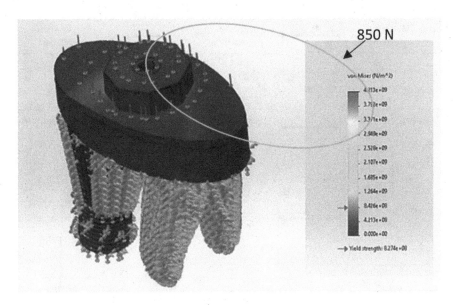

FIGURE 5.8   Static-Stress analysis result of MRDI assembly on SOLIDWORKS.

were removed from the construct plate using wire electrical discharge machining. Figure 5.9 shows a process flow for the printing of MRDI.

5.4   FABRICATION OF TIBIA BONE FROM MEDICAL IMAGING DATA TO A 3D PRINTED ANATOMICAL MODEL

AM technology is now rapidly emerging and evolving from a prototype fabrication technique into a real-product manufacturing technology in multidisciplines (Boparai et al., 2021a, 2021b, 2022a, 2022b, 2016). The tibia bone is one of the longest bones in canine species and is important for movement function and helps with weight bearing. The tibia bone articulates proximally concerning the femur bone, the tarsus distally, and the fibula both proximally and distally on its lateral side. The tibia bone act as a support for many nearby muscles and fractures are relatively common in canine patients. In young dogs, the most common reason for tibia fractures is trauma. Tibia bone fractures are diaphyseal. Internal and external fixation has been used in surgical practice to repair tibia bone fractures. It is reported that fracture healing by rigid fixation techniques involves fewer complications and an increase in healing (Johnson et al., 1989, 1996; Palmer et al., 1992). Fracture of the cranial cruciate ligament in canine patients leads to unusual movement of the tibia and extra rotation to the knee joint internally, which may cause osteoarthritis (Elkins et al., 1991; Vasseur and Berry, 1992). Bibliographic analysis for the keywords "tibia bone fracture medical imaging" and the research gap analysis are respectively shown in Figures 5.10 and 5.11.

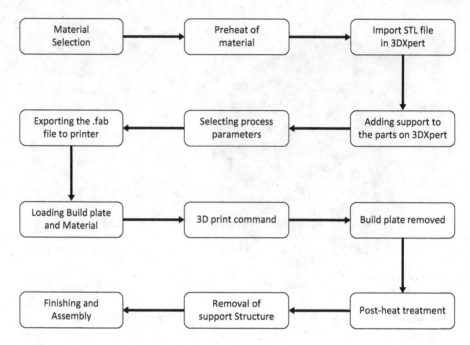

FIGURE 5.9 Flow chart for fabrication of MRDI parts on DMLS.

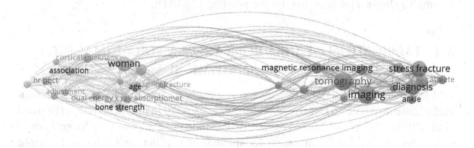

FIGURE 5.10 Bibliographic analysis for the keywords "tibia bone fracture medical imaging".

Since the discovery of medical imaging modalities (X-ray) (Roentgen, 1895), their use in medical treatment has evolved from 2D-3D radiographs to 4D radiographs. The emergence of newer technologies has enhanced the abilities of medical residents to perform successful surgical procedures. Substantial improvements in diagnostic image quality have been seen with reduced image acquisition time. The development of ultrasonography (ultrasound) in the 1950s established the use of sound waves. In addition to this, the use of thermal imaging in the 1950s highlighted the use of temperature screening to generate diagnostic image data. The magnetic resonance imaging (MRI) technique developed in 1971 revealed the use

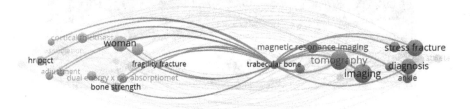

FIGURE 5.11 Research gap analysis for "trabecular bone".

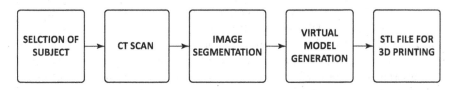

FIGURE 5.12 Framework to use medical imaging data to reconstruct the bone model.

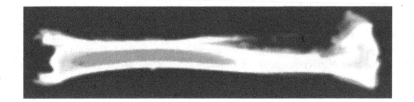

FIGURE 5.13 Image acquisition of the tibia bone.

of magnetic resonance to improve image resolution. The development of the computed tomography (CT) machine permitted the generation of 3-dimensional (3D) medical images which may be further manipulated to plan surgical treatment. The generic framework to use medical imaging data to reconstruct the bone model is shown in Figure 5.12.

In this case study, CT scan data of a tibia bone stored in DICOM format was used for reconstructing the virtual model of the tibia bone. In this study the open-source software "RadiANT" DICOM viewer was used to convert medical imaging databases and surface reconstruction. The non-contrast computed tomography (NCCT) medical image information was taken from cadaver specimens of the tibia, and bone was acquired from CT scan X-ray (Siemens SOMATOM scope observer model) with the spiral acquisition process. The interpreted medical imaging data can be converted into a virtual CAD model and Standard Tessellation Language (STL format) for AM (Figures 5.13 and 5.14).

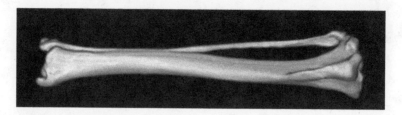

FIGURE 5.14   Reconstructed tibia bone.

5.5   SUMMARY

This chapter highlights a case study for orthopedics and dentistry using medical imaging data. The presented work showcases the procedure to fabricate an in-house-prepared, low-cost MRDI prototype for a canine by 3D printing. It may be used effectively for the biomedical practices of patients. Similarly, the workflow to prepare the STL file for 3D printing of a tibia bone has been outlined. The work reveals the importance of both areas (veterinary and orthopedics) using medical imaging and demonstrates how it may help to obtain better solutions for preoperative surgical planning and reconstructive surgery cases.

REFERENCES

Boparai, K.S., Kumar, A., Kumar, A., Aman, A. and Singh, S., 2021a. Nanomaterial in additive manufacturing for energy storage applications. In C.M. Hussain (Ed.), *Handbook of Polymer Nanocomposites for Industrial Applications* (pp. 529–543). Amsterdam, Netherlands: Elsevier.

Boparai, K.S. and Kumara, A., 2021b. Thermosetting polymers as scaffold applications. In *Encyclopedia of Materials: Plastics and Polymers* (Vol. 1, pp. 588–595). Amsterdam, Netherlands: Elsevier Inc. https://doi.org/10.1016/B978-0-12-820352-1.00110-3.

Boparai, K.S., Kumar, A. and Singh, R., 2022a. On characterization of rechargeable, flexible electrochemical energy storage device. In R. Singh (Ed.), *4D Printing* (pp. 67–88). Amsterdam, Netherlands: Elsevier Inc.

Boparai, K.S., Kumar, A. and Singh, R., 2022b. Primary and secondary melt processing for plastics. In R. Singh and R. Kumar (Eds.), *Additive Manufacturing for Plastic Recycling* (pp. 51–65). Boca Raton, FL: CRC Press.

Boparai, K.S., Singh, R. and Singh, H., 2016. Development of rapid tooling using fused deposition modeling: A review. *Rapid Prototyping Journal*, 22(2), pp. 281–299. https://doi.org/10.1108/RPJ-04-2014-0048.

Box, V.H., Sukotjo, C., Knoernschild, K.L., Campbell, S.D. and Afshari, F.S., 2018. Patient-reported and clinical outcomes of implant-supported fixed complete dental prostheses: A comparison of metal acrylic, milled zirconia, and retrievable crown prostheses. *Journal of Oral Implantology*, 44(1), pp. 51–61.

Coffman, C., Visser, C., Soukup, J. and Peak, M., 2019. Crowns and prosthodontics. In H.B. Lobprise and R. Johnathon (Eds.), *Wiggs's Vet Dent* (pp. 387–410). Hoboken, NJ: John Wiley & Sons, Inc. https://doi.org/10.1002/9781118816219.ch18.

Elkins, A.D., Pechman, R., Kearney, M.T. and Herron, M., 1991. A retrospective study evaluating the degree of degenerative joint disease in the stifle joint of dogs following surgical repair of anterior cruciate ligament rupture. *Journal of the American Animal Hospital Association*, 27(5), pp. 533–540.

Gebhardt, A., Schmidt, F.M., Hötter, J.S., Sokalla, W. and Sokalla, P., 2010. Additive manufacturing by selective laser melting the realizer desktop machine and its application for the dental industry. *Physics Procedia*, 5, pp. 543–549.

Johnson, A.L., Kneller, S.K. and Weigel, R.M., 1989. Radial and tibial fracture repair with external skeletal fixation: Effects of fracture type, reduction, and complications on healing. *Veterinary Surgery*, 18(5), pp. 367–372.

Johnson, A.L., Seitz, S.E., Smith, C.W., Johnson, J.M. and Schaeffer, D.J., 1996. Closed reduction and type-II external fixation of comminuted fractures of the radius and tibia in dogs: 23 Cases (1990–1994). *Journal of the American Veterinary Medical Association*, 209(8), pp. 1445–1448.

Li, C., Pisignano, D., Zhao, Y. and Xue, J., 2020. Advances in medical applications of additive manufacturing. *Engineering*, 6(11), pp. 1222–1231.

Novakov, T., Jackson, M.J., Robinson, G.M., Ahmed, W. and Phoenix, D.A., 2017. Laser sintering of metallic medical materials—A review. *The International Journal of Advanced Manufacturing Technology*, 93(5), pp. 2723–2752.

Palmer, R.H., Hulse, D.A., Hyman, W.A. and Palmer, D.R., 1992. Principles of bone healing and biomechanics of external skeletal fixation. *Veterinary Clinics of North America: Small Animal Practice*, 22(1), pp. 45–68.

Pradhan, S.R., Singh, R. and Banwait, S.S., 2021. On crown fabrication in prosthetic dentistry of veterinary patients: A review. *Advances in Materials and Processing Technologies*. https://doi.org/10.1080/2374068X.2021.1970991.

Sames, W.J., List, F.A., Pannala, S., Dehoff, R.R. and Babu, S.S., 2016. The metallurgy and processing science of metal additive manufacturing. *International Materials Reviews*, 61(5), pp. 315–360.

Singh, R., Sharma, R. and Ranjan, N., 2017. Four-dimensional printing for clinical dentistry. *Encyclopedia of Smart Materials*, 1, pp. 329–355. https://doi.org/10.1016/B978-0-12-803581-8.10167-5.

Vasseur, P.B. and Berry, C.R., 1992. Progression of stifle osteoarthrosis following reconstruction of the cranial cruciate ligament in 21 dogs. *Journal of the American Animal Hospital Association*, 28(2), pp. 129–136.

6 In-house Development of Smart Materials for 4D Printing

Vinay Kumar, Rupinder Singh, and
Inderpreet Singh Ahuja

CONTENTS

6.1 INTRODUCTION

In the past three decades, the significant influence of smart materials has been reported by researchers for advanced manufacturing, structural engineering, and biomedical applications. The changes and improvements that occurred in the processing of various materials (e.g., petroleum and petroleum products) increased demand for reliable, durable, and cost-effective mass consumer products (Tomlinson and Bullough, 1998). The energy-efficient micro-devices prepared for cell-mimicking of molecular assemblies and for detecting pathogenic agents have also been regarded as smart materials for biosensing applications (Song et al., 2002). The sol-gel process has been reported as a smart method for the preparation of various smart materials since this approach allows the fabrication of organically modified materials whose molecular structure can be designed according to requirements (Rao and Dave, 2002). Studies that highlighted the bending response in polymer-metal composites for hand prostheses, due to electro-active properties (Biddiss and Chau 2006), intelligent filtration properties in hyper-branched polymers (Seiler 2006), and

DOI: 10.1201/9781003205531-6

self-assembly properties in light-sensitive thermoplastics (Seki 2006), can be considered as smart materials prepared for useful biomedical applications. The investigations performed by the researchers on the recent synthesis of smart ceramics, polymer blends, shape-memory alloys, and ferromagnetic materials, highlighted the role of smart materials in the study of aquatic animals, robotics, non-destructive testing, one-way programmed porous substrates, and membranes, etc. (Schwartz 2008). The utilization of smart composite structure materials has been reported as being a novel approach for supporting structural health-monitoring activities (Epaarachchi and Kahandawa, 2016). The integration of such materials with advanced monitoring solutions may be used to restore and rehabilitate the valuable cultural heritage of the world.

The use of smart materials in processes such as 3D printing, to prepare the function prototypes of programmable materials (polymer blends or composites) for 4D application areas such as clinical dentistry and veterinary sciences, has indicated that novel, cost-effective, and customized 4D solutions may be delivered for the betterment of future generations (Singh et al., 2017). The literature survey reveals that 3D/4D printing has emerged as a novel and acceptable approach to manufacturing cost-effective industrial products, sensors, and actuators for devices. The 4D printing of polymers is now being explored widely for advanced space exploration, and biomedical and structural applications, by utilizing smart materials that possess shape-memory or programming properties. Table 6.1 highlights the various key terms investigated by the researchers (for the past three decades) with regard to the preparation and utilization of smart materials and their 3D/4D printing applications (based on the "web of knowledge" database).

Out of 504 research terms reported on smart materials, 77 highly reported keywords (in terms of occurrence and relevance) (Table 6.1) outlined that the commercially available smart materials (ceramics- and composite-based) are reportedly very costly for the desired application in developing countries. Nevertheless, little has been reported on the in-house development of smart materials for 3D and 4D printing applications. The review of recent advances in 3D/4D printing technology and applications, and the utilization of recycled materials as composites for the repair of heritage structures with shape-memory polymers, has outlined the importance of efficient processes to manufacture suitable smart materials (Zhang et al., 2019, Singh and Kumar, 2020, Falahati et al., 2020, Akbar et al., 2022). Based on Table 6.1, the interlinking of various research areas such as 3D printing technology, design of smart materials, optimization of processing parameters, and characteristic analysis of 4D printed materials are shown in Figure 6.1.

Figure 6.1 also outlines the process flow involved in the 4D printing of smart materials. The process starts with designing and simulating materials to prepare smart materials, followed by parametric optimization.

Based on optimized results mechanical, thermal, and other characteristics are ascertained to finally fabricate the 3D/4D printed product for the desired application. Three-dimensionally printed smart energy storage devices (Kumar and Kumar, 2020), textile-based sensors (Liu et al., 2022), and thermoplastic composites with 4D capabilities (Kumar et al., 2022a, 2022b) have been explored by following such

TABLE 6.1
List of Reported Research Terms with Regard to Smart Materials and 4D Printing

Id	Term	Occurrences	Relevance Score
1	3D printed structure	4	0.7207
2	4D bioprinting	6	2.2119
3	4D printing concept	4	1.5484
4	4D printing method	9	0.8702
5	Active material	11	0.5135
6	Advanced material	6	1.2089
7	Application field	4	0.9817
8	Artificial muscle	9	0.5998
9	Battery	5	0.6701
10	Biocompatibility	9	0.5073
11	Biomedical application	14	0.7203
12	Biomedical device	14	0.571
13	Biomedical engineering	5	1.1878
14	Bio-mimetic 4D printing	4	1.5792
15	Bioprinting	8	1.9642
16	Bone	5	1.7279
17	Carbon nano-tube	7	0.9015
18	Conductive material	4	0.8859
19	Digital light processing	7	1.1556
20	Deposition modeling	10	0.87
21	Deformation behavior	4	1.1828
22	Deployable structure	6	0.6848
23	Direct ink writing	5	1.0949
24	Drug delivery	8	0.9063
25	Dynamic response	5	1.0335
26	Dynamic structure	6	1.273
27	Electrical conductivity	4	1.0049
28	Environmental stimulus	6	0.6932
29	Excellent shape-memory performance	5	1.4003
30	Exposure	9	0.5998
31	Extension	4	1.9449
32	External stimulation	5	1.2396
33	Extrusion	7	0.5074
34	Flexible electronic	4	1.0235
35	Fourth dimension	13	0.7521
36	Framework	12	1.6499
37	Fundamental	5	1.9652
38	Fundamental understanding	4	1.6497
39	Future application	8	0.8351

(Continued)

TABLE 6.1 (CONTINUED)
List of Reported Research Terms with Regard to Smart
Materials and 4D Printing

Id	Term	Occurrences	Relevance Score
40	Future direction	4	1.3003
41	Innovative technology	4	1.4569
42	Mechanical behavior	7	0.9187
43	Mechanical property	27	0.5913
44	Mechanical strength	5	1.1159
45	Medical field	5	1.4418
46	Multifunctional material	5	0.985
47	Multiple materials	5	1.124
48	Natural material	4	1.1279
49	Novel technology	5	0.8712
50	Nozzle temperature	4	1.1491
51	Origami	7	0.692
52	Polylactic acid	11	0.7409
53	Polymer material	7	0.767
54	Polyurethane	6	0.8878
55	Printable smart material	5	1.0572
56	Process parameter	15	0.7886
57	Programming	18	0.3673
58	Prototype	9	0.5984
59	Rapid development	5	0.907
60	Regenerative medicine	4	1.6228
61	Reinforcement	5	0.7267
62	Responsive polymer	7	0.4155
63	Responsiveness	10	0.4268
64	Review article	8	1.3722
65	Selective laser melting	5	1.3394
66	Self assembly	4	1.9566
67	Self-folding	5	0.9767
68	Shape-memory polymer composite	5	1.1044
69	Shape-memory property	13	0.6507
70	Shape programming	4	0.6152
71	Shape recovery	12	0.7236
72	Shape-recovery process	7	0.963
73	Stereolithography	6	0.9527
74	Target shape	5	1.1523
75	Temporal dimension	4	1.0363
76	Temporary shape	7	0.8052
77	Tissue engineering	21	0.9693

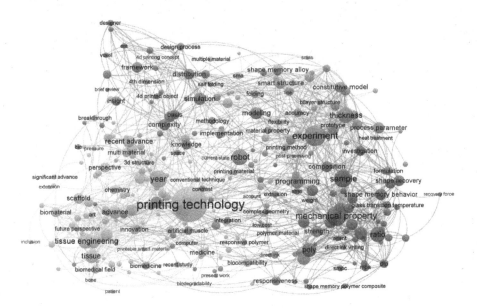

FIGURE 6.1 Web of key research areas for smart materials and 4D printing.

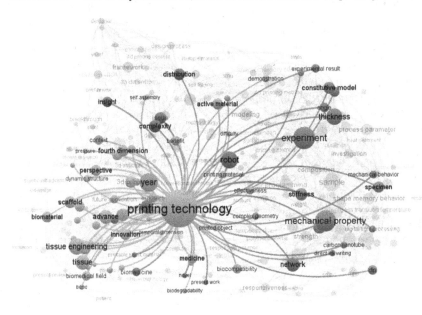

FIGURE 6.2 Influence of design and simulation of smart materials for 4D printing.

methodology for 4D printing. Figure 6.2 shows the effect of design insight, material distribution on various properties, and optimized results for successful 4D printing. The studies reported on parametric optimization of 4D-capable smart materials (such as polylactic acid (PLA), polybutylene succinate (PBS), acrylonitrile butadiene

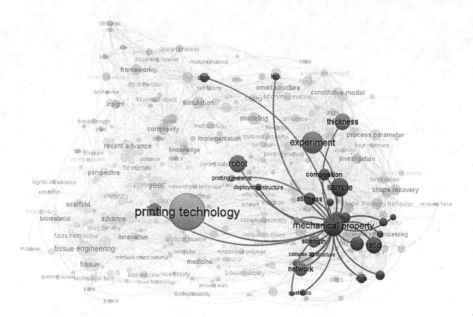

FIGURE 6.3 Effect of parametric optimization for acceptable 4D printing.

styrene (ABS)), and hybrid filaments for various printing technologies, are supported by Figure 6.3 (Lin et al., 2022; Kumar et al., 2020a). This indicates the significant effect of experimental observations and process parameter optimization on ascertaining acceptable mechanical strength for different additive manufacturing-based manufacturing technologies for proposed 4D applications (Kumar et al., 2022c).

The investigations performed on rheological, thermal, mechanical, electric, magnetic, optical, morphological, and piezoelectric properties of polymer composites matrices (having ABS, polyvinylidene fluoride (PVDF), polyvinyl chloride (PVC), and polypropylene (PP)), for sensor (Jain et al., 2022; Kumar et al., 2020b) and smart repair works, have highlighted that an appropriate processing route of smart materials is required to impart 4D characteristics into the composite for the desired results (Ranjan et al., 2021; Kumar et al., 2022d). Similarly, Figure 6.4 shows the successful impact of analysis on 3D/4D printing of smart polymeric materials such as low-density polyethylene (LDPE)-bakelite blends, PVDF-Mn-doped ZnO composites that have been reported for biomedical applications, and online health monitoring of electronic devices (Kumar et al., 2022e; Fu et al., 2022; Kumar et al., 2021a).

6.2 LITERATURE GAP

The studies reported on the preparation of various smart material matrices such as blends, alloys, composites, ceramics, and compounds for 4D applications have outlined that chemical-assisted mechanical blending is a novel approach to preparing self-acting–type polymer-based composites. Further, multi-material 3D printing of

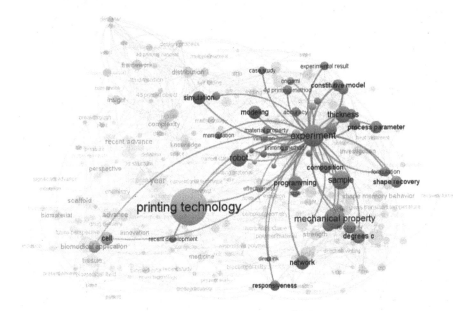

FIGURE 6.4 Role of characterization and optimization in 4D printing.

such electro-active, self-healing composites may be performed to maintain heritage structures (Sharma et al., 2021; Kumar et al., 2021b, 2012c). But hitherto, little has been reported on the use of such smart materials based on 4D properties for the development of customized solutions in the case of patients facing bone fractures in the hip joint. The present study reports the path that may be followed to utilize the self-expansion and self-contraction properties of thermoplastic composites for the treatment of hip joints, especially in those cases in which the bones of patients degraded with time due to age factors or poor immunity. Finally, a framework for the fabrication of smart/rapid tooling to be used in total hip arthroplasty (THA) (having 4D capabilities) is detailed in this work.

6.3   ROLE OF 3D TECHNOLOGY IN THA

The computer-technology–assisted 3D models and structures of multiple images can be used to perform surgical activities such as THA. Also, for navigation assistance and preoperative surgical planning of THA, 3D scanning is performed. For typical surgical procedures in hip-joint replacement, THA, and osteotomy, 3D scanning and finite element analysis (FEA)-based outcomes can be used to prepare 3D printed models of damage zones to support the surgeon in successful operation/surgery. Figure 6.5 shows the integration of 3D technologies such as scanning, mimicking, modeling, printing, etc. with orthopedics to prepare a digital platform for surgical applications. The digital orthopedic system equipped with digital anatomy, 3D printing, FEA, and navigational, virtual, and robotic surgery features, can be used to save time and for cost-effective surgery.

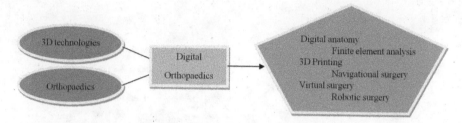

FIGURE 6.5 Digital orthopedic platform and its applications.

The advantage of digital orthopedics lies in the management of surgical procedures and supporting orthopedists during preoperative decisions, intraoperative manipulation, and post-operative management. Digital orthopedics technology also includes virtual operation training, virtual operative planning, rapid prototype-assisted operations, computer-assisted navigation in operations, etc. Before surgery, all instruments should be reviewed to ensure they are present and working properly. Then the appropriate osteotomy guide, based on preoperative templating, is chosen. The silver guide is for standard offset implants and the gold guide is for high-offset implants. The ante-version handle is then threaded into the osteotomy guide. If the template is based on the femoral head location, assembly of the sliding head guide to the osteotomy guide is performed (Höwell et al., 2004). Based on preoperative templating, alignment of the sliding head guide with the appropriate stem-size laser marked on the osteotomy guide is performed. Then the assembled guide is placed against the femur, aligning the femoral head with the sliding head guide. The femoral neck resection can then be marked using electrocautery. If templating is based on using the tip of the greater trochanter, the sliding head guide is not needed. A spinal needle is used to find the trochanter tip. An appropriate osteotomy guide (standard or high offset) is placed against the femur and located using the distance from the tip of the greater trochanter to the top of the prosthesis. The femoral neck resection can then be marked using electrocautery. Preparation of the acetabulum is done if acetabular reconstruction is required (Parratte and Argenson, 2007).

6.4   CONVENTIONAL METHODS OF THA

6.4.1   Step 1: Femoral Canal Fabrication

The first step followed for THA surgeries includes the preparation of the femoral canal. Figure 6.6 shows the steps involved in the conventional THA process. The box osteotome and canal finder are used for initial entry into the femoral canal. After this, broach assembly and disassembly operations are performed. For assembly of the broach to the broach handle, placement of the broach post in the clamp is done in the first stage. The thumb is used to lock the clamp onto the broach. A modular ante-version handle can be assembled to the broach handle to provide version control. Then the broach from the broach handle is disassembled by lifting the lever to release the handle from the broach post.

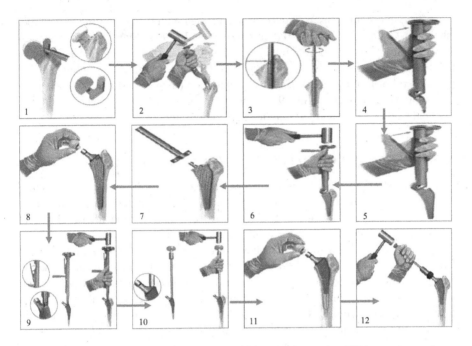

FIGURE 6.6   Conventional steps in technique for broaching during THA.

6.4.2   STEP 2: FEMORAL BROACHING

The femoral broaching procedure is started along the axis of the femur with the starter broach. Sequential broaching is then carried out to the ideal stem-size using valgus force on the stem handle. Taking care to preserve the greater trochanter, the starter broach can be used to rasp laterally beneath the greater trochanter. The stability of the broach is checked rotationally, medially, and laterally. Broaching is stopped only when stability is achieved. It is important to maintain broach rotation due to the rectangular geometry of the implant (Kennedy et al., 1998).

6.4.3   STEP 3: CALCAR PREPARATION

With the final broach fully seated, the broach handle is removed. Calcar reamer is placed over the post of the broach and the femoral neck is machined, ensuring alignment to avoid femur fracture. In the trial reduction step, the standard or high-offset trial neck (as determined by templating) is then placed onto the broach post using forceps. The trial femoral head of the desired diameter is selected and +0 neck-length and placed onto the trial neck. Then the hip is reduced and leg-length is re-measured and compared against previous measurements recorded from preoperative templating or leg-length before dislocation. Adjustments in neck-length and/or offset can be made at this time if trialing for a polar or bipolar trial, according to the appropriate technique for the selected device. After assembly and disassembly of the broach, the stem is inserted into the seat created with the help of the broach tool (shown in 12 steps in Figure 6.6) (Schmalzried et al., 1994). Step 1 shows the femoral osteotomy process followed by femoral canal preparation (Steps 2 and 3). Step 4 involves the starter broach assembly process, then the broach disassembly (Step 5) and femoral broaching (Step 6). Calcar preparation (Step7), trial reduction (Step 8), and stem insertion of rigid (Step 9) and non-rigid inserts (Step 10) are performed for the final trial (Step 11) and femoral head assembly (Step 12).

6.5   4D PRINTED CUSTOMIZED SOLUTION FOR THA

The present status of THA cases around the globe indicates the exponential increase in developed as well as in developing nations. The aging population, sedentary lifestyles, booming economies, and the high cost of living demand the development of smart 4D solutions to prepare a bio-compatible and customizable broach as a 3D printed smart rapid tool to resolve THA cases cost-effectively in less time. Cost-effective solutions may be affordable to a wide range of patients. Although traditional total hip-replacement surgery has a high success rate, the customizable-solution approach not only speeds up the surgery and enhances surgical precision but also makes post-operative recovery faster than before. The custom-designed cutting guides and instruments allow orthopedic surgeons to precisely position the knee implant during surgery, avoiding misalignment which can potentially lead to early implant failure. Figure 6.7 shows the proposed work methodology to prepare a multi-material 4D printed smart tool as a solution for THA.

In particular, it has been proposed that instead of metal, a polymer-composite structure may be used. The rasp is intended to be manufactured inexpensively, making it suitable for single use and thereby making cleaning and sterilization of the used rasp unnecessary. The rasp includes a connecting section for connecting the rasp to an impact tool. Other devices, comprised entirely of a polymer, have also been proposed. The tailor-made/patient-specific applications of this work lie in the manufacturing of different size broaches with the help of multi-material 3D printing. The newly developed rapid tooling may be included in the dedicated instruments category. So, the present work may help reduce complications by appropriate selection of 3D/4D customized tooling.

6.6   ROLE OF SMART THERMOPLASTIC COMPOSITES IN 4D APPLICATIONS

A problem with the non-metallic tool is that it does not have the same rigidity as a metallic one. During the surgical process, a broach or rasp is subjected to high stress as it impacts the bone. Plastic broaches or rasps are less suited to withstanding these forces. So, rigid metallic broaches are used as they do not yield when pressed against the bone that is to be removed. Smart, 3D printed thermoplastic composites with acceptable strength can fulfill the need for an alternative approach to reduce the cost and weight of medical devices such as broaches or rasps, in which the sturdiness and

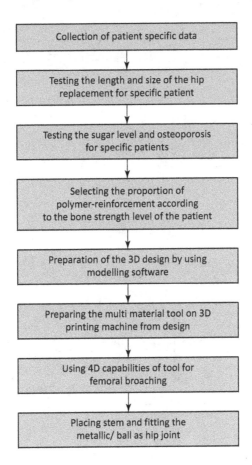

FIGURE 6.7   Work methodology.

rigidity of earlier solid metal devices may be retained. A device such as a broach or a rasp having a hard polymer central member surrounded by an outer portion comprising a polymer and reinforcement is shown in Figure 6.8. It is relatively light in weight, more durable, and can better withstand impaction forces involved in bone removal (for instance, during the preparation of the medullary cavity of a patient to receive an implant) as compared to earlier devices comprised of solid metal. According to the patient's sugar level and osteoporosis, the reinforcement levels of the outer portions of the tool may be varied. Figure 6.9 provides a complete picture of the proposed broach tool. The conventional broach tool in surgeries is used for rendering the size of the femur. This broaching procedure is known as femoral broaching. This includes the broaching of the femur with various differentially sized broaches and thus may be known as sequential broaching.

The multi-material 3D printed smart broach tool for femoral broaching of the bone for total hip replacement can be fabricated from pure and reinforced bio-compatible polymer. The pure polymer may be used as a central member and reinforced

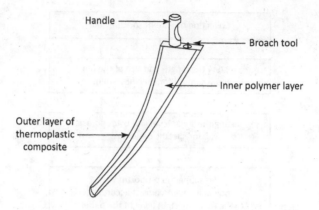

FIGURE 6.8   2D sketch of proposed broach tool.

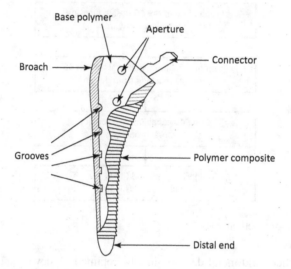

FIGURE 6.9   Different aspects of multi-material 3D printed smart broach tool.

polymer composite on the outer side, that outer layer with a rough surface contributed to the removal of the bone particle to make size compatible with the stem to be
used. The ridges or grooves can act to grip the polymer of the outer portion during
the impaction of the device. Therefore, once aligned along a direction transverse
to a longitudinal axis of the device, they optimally withstand the forces associated
with impaction of the device. A connector may be provided at the proximal end
of the device for attachment to a handle. The connector can be formed from the
proximal end of the pure polymer central member allowing for a robust connection to the handle. The connector can be a male- or a female-type connector. The
distal end of the pure polymer central member extends through the outer portion to
form the tip of the device. The patient suffering from osteoporosis (i.e., degradation of bone with age and time) can be treated using the smart tool. Persons with

osteoporosis have different levels of bone strength. So, the tooling needed for the femoral broaching of such patients may differ according to the size of the implant, the strength, and the broaching capacity of both the bone and the tool. In the proposed smart tool, the broaching capacity, size, and strength of the tool can be varied along the circumference and length of the tool by adding different proportions of reinforcements of ceramic, magnetic, or electrically conducting nano-particles for 4D features. 4D programming-based performance standards play a much greater role in joint replacement because the performance of the tool may be varied according to patient-specific data.

6.7   FABRICATION OF MULTI-MATERIAL 3D PRINTED SMART BROACH TOOL

The multi-material 3D printed smart broach tool with 4D features based on self-contraction and self elongation can be prepared with bio-compatible material such as PVC, PVDF, and polylactic acid (PLA) along with the reinforcement like Mn-doped ZnO, $CaCO_3$, chitosan, hydroxyapatite, almond skin, and Al_2O_3. It has been reported that electro-active, magnetic, bio-compatible, piezoelectricity, and one-way programming-based 4D features can be induced in the multi-material printed composite matrix by the application of external electric and magnetic fields (Kumar et al., 2021c; Kumar et al., 2022d). An alternative route for making the multi-material, customized, economical, and lightweight reinforced polymer-based surgical broach may be established with such smart materials. The proposed methodology will allow a surgeon to use a custom-made broach on the spot for a specific patient with the help of 3D printing. This will also help in reducing the cost of surgery to some extent and also reduce or even eliminate the waiting time for the arrival of the tool. Further, this will reduce treatment time for the THR, thus reducing the pain level of the patient because there is no need to use undersized broaches. This technology may also be used for other orthopedic surgeries such as total knee replacement (TKR). The steps listed below may be followed to fabricate a multi-material 3D printed smart broach tool with 4D capabilities:

- Investigating the mechanical blending and chemical-assisted mechanical blending approaches of material processing for ascertaining acceptable rheological, mechanical, thermal, and 4D properties in the composite.
- Preparation of smart 3D printer filament wire for a fused deposition modeling machine (FDM) from bio-compatible composite-based polymer matrix (such as PLA, PVDF, and PVC as matrix material and Mn-doped ZnO, $CaCO_3$, chitosan, hydroxyapatite, almond skin, Al_2O_3 as reinforcement).
- Multi-material 3D printing of composites to prepare the surgical rapid tooling that possesses biocompatibility, mechanical strength, and 4D properties.
- Investigating the 4D-based customizable features such as self-healing, self-elongation, and self-contraction in the 3D printed tool to prepare an economical and lightweight surgical broach.

- In vitro and corrosion analysis of the smart broach to check the suitability, biocompatibility, and degradation rate of the developed broach.
- Analysis of mechanical strain, and the thermal, electrical, magnetic, and morphological properties of the developed tooling by piezoelectric, dynamic mechanical analysis (DMA), Fourier transformed infrared (FTIR), X-ray diffraction (XRD), and scattered electron microscopy (SEM) analysis.
- Performing process capability analysis (of the proposed route) for fabrication of surgical tooling to develop a customized broach or rasp that can be used specifically by the dimensions of the body part of the patient on which replacement has to be performed, with the help of 3D printing.

The application of a smart 3D broach with customization features lies in shaping the bone as per the condition/fitness of the patient's damaged bone. Reinforcement with a high response towards external stimulus may contribute to imparting 4D properties to a bio-compatible matrix-based polymer composite for the desired action. Realizations of this invention can provide a device such as a broach or a rasp for use in orthopedic surgery. In particular, the device will be used to remove bone during orthopedic surgery. The broach will also be used to remove bone from the medullary canal itself, to prepare the femur for the installation of an appropriately sized femoral implant. The composite-based multi-material 3D printed tool with self-healing capabilities possesses acceptable structural strength and rigidity, while the outer portion of the device, which comprises a self-actuating polymer composite, can be molded around the central member, allowing the cutting or rasping features of the device (e.g., teeth, ribs, or ridges) to be formed. Overall, such tools and devices can retain a degree of rigidity that approximates the rigidity and sturdiness of commercially available broaches or rasps, along with low-cost and reduced-weight features. Such low-cost tools may also be used as single-use devices that can be discarded after a surgical procedure, thereby avoiding the need to clean and sterilize the device for subsequent further use. The recyclability of the base polymer matrix allows fabrication of a new tool after recycling. While three-dimensionally printing the new tool, the outer shape and dimensions of the broach (known as art) can be chosen to substantially match the shape of the stem of the femoral implant that is to be inserted into the medullar canal. Therefore, customization is possible in every manufacturing cycle.

The proposed composite-based smart customizable tool is highly beneficial for patients and surgeons who are involved in hip-replacement surgeries. 3D printing provides design and fabrication flexibility whereas the material processing routes may be selected as per the desired cost of manufacturing the final product. Although devices made entirely of polymer, polymer ceramics composites, and thermoplastic composite matrices are lighter and more economical to manufacture, surgeons typically prefer devices such as broaches or rasps that have the rigidity of solid metal. During a surgical procedure, the surgeon can select an appropriately sized broach by the dimensions of the femoral implant. Also, as is known in the art, a surgeon may begin a bone-removal procedure using a relatively small broach or rasp and subsequently use larger devices of a similar kind as the opening in the medullary canal is increased in size. In this regard, patients with hip dimensions not matching with the surgical tool will be the target beneficiaries. Customized broaches can be made with the help of 3D printing on the spot, according to the dimensions of the hip that has to be replaced. This technology will simplify the procedure of total hip replacements by providing the surgical instrument kit based on the leg-length and other dimensions of the body.

6.8 SUMMARY

The in-house smart thermoplastic composite prepared by reinforcing stimulus-responsive elements for 3D/4D printing applications may be used effectively for biomedical practices such as THA and TKR. Compared to commercially available solutions for THA, the proposed customizable solution prepared by multi-material 3D printing of composite structures may be used as a recyclable, economic, and cost-effective solution for treating THA. The self-expanding and self-contracting–based 4D printing properties of the fabricated solution will be useful in the self-adjustment of multi-material 3D printed tools to accommodate uneven disorders present in the bone (due to osteoporosis). As a result of such features, complications in the surgical process may be avoided.

6.9 REFERENCES

Akbar, I., El Hadrouz, M., El Mansori, M. and Lagoudas, D., 2022. Toward enabling manufacturing paradigm of 4D printing of shape memory materials: Open literature review. *European Polymer Journal*, 168, p. 111106.

Biddiss, E. and Chau, T., 2006. Electroactive polymeric sensors in hand prostheses: Bending response of an ionic polymer-metal composite. *Medical Engineering and Physics*, 28(6), pp. 568–578.

Epaarachchi, J.A. and Kahandawa, G.C., 2016. *Structural Health Monitoring Technologies and Next-Generation Smart Composite Structures* (1st ed.). CRC Press. https://doi.org /10.1201/9781315373492.

Falahati, M., Ahmadvand, P., Safaee, S., Chang, Y.C., Lyu, Z., Chen, R., Li, L. and Lin, Y., 2020. Smart polymers and nanocomposites for 3D and 4D printing. *Materials Today*, 40, pp. 215–245.

Fu, P., Li, H., Gong, J., Fan, Z., Smith, A.T., Shen, K., Khalfalla, T.O., Huang, H., Qian, X., McCutcheon, J.R. and Sun, L., 2022. 4D printing of polymeric materials: Techniques, materials, and prospects. *Progress in Polymer Science*, 126, p. 101506.

Höwell, J.R., Masri, B.A. and Duncan, C.P., 2004. Minimally invasive versus standard incision anterolateral hip replacement: A comparative study. *Orthopedic Clinics of North America*, 35(2), pp. 153–162.

Jain, C., Dhaliwal, B.S. and Singh, R., 2022. On 3D-printed acrylonitrile butadiene styrene-based sensors: Rheological, mechanical, morphological, radio frequency, and 4D capabilities. *Journal of Materials Engineering and Performance*, pp. 1–15. https://doi.org /10.1007/s11665-022-06884-4.

Kennedy, J.G., Rogers, W.B., Soffe, K.E., Sullivan, R.J., Griffen, D.G. and Sheehan, L.J., 1998. Effect of acetabular component orientation on recurrent dislocation, pelvic osteolysis, polyethylene wear, and component migration. *Journal of Arthroplasty*, 13(5), pp. 530–534.

Kumar, R. and Kumar, P., 2020a. Li-doped ZnO nanoparticles reinforcement in PVDF ther-moplastic matrix for 3D printing of charge storage devices. Reference module in mate-rials science and materials engineering. https://doi.org/10.1016/B978-0-12-820352-1 .00029-8.

Kumar, R., Pandey, A.K., Singh, R. and Kumar, V., 2020b. On Nano, polypyrrole, and carbon nanotube reinforced PVDF for 3D printing applications: Rheological, thermal, elec-trical, mechanical, morphological characterization. *Journal of Composite Materials*, 54(29), pp. 4677–4689.

Kumar, R., Singh, R., Kumar, V. and Kumar, P., 2021a. On Mn-doped ZnO nanoparticles reinforced in PVDF matrix for fused filament fabrication: Mechanical, thermal, mor-phological, and 4D properties. *Journal of Manufacturing Processes*, 62, pp. 817–832.

Kumar, S., Singh, R. and Singh, M., 2021b. Multi-material 3D printed PLA/PA6-TiO2 composite matrix: Rheological, thermal, tensile, morphological, and 4D capabilities. *Advances in Materials and Processing Technologies*, pp. 1–19. https://doi.org/10.1080 /2374068X.2021.1912527.

Kumar, S., Singh, R., Singh, A.P. and Wei, Y., 2022e. Case study for the development of a hybrid composite structure of thermosetting and thermoplastics. In R. Singh and R. Kumar (Ed.), *Additive Manufacturing for Plastic Recycling* (pp. 141–157). Boca Raton, FL: CRC Press.

Kumar, V., Singh, R. and Ahuja, I.P.S., 2020a. Effect of extrusion parameters on primary recycled ABS: Mechanical, rheological, morphological, and thermal properties. *Materials Research Express*, 7(1), p. 015208.

Kumar, V., Singh, R. and Ahuja, I.S., 2021c. On 3D printing of electro-active PVDF-graphene and Mn-doped ZnO nanoparticle-based composite as a self-healing repair solution for heritage structures. *Proceedings of the Institution of Mechanical Engineers, Part B*, 236(8), pp. 1141–1154. https://doi.org/10.1177/09544054211060912.

Kumar, V., Singh, R. and Ahuja, I.S., 2022a. On the programming of polyvinylidene fluo-ride–limestone composite for four-dimensional printing applications in heritage struc-tures. *Proceedings of the Institution of Mechanical Engineers, Part L*, 236(2), pp. 319–333.

Kumar, V., Singh, R. and Ahuja, I.P.S., 2022b. On 4D capabilities of chemical assisted mechanical blended ABS-Nano graphene composite matrix. *Materials Today: Proceedings*, 48, pp. 952–957.

Kumar, V., Singh, R. and Ahuja, I.S., 2022c. Hybrid feedstock filament processing for the preparation of composite structures in heritage repair. In R. Singh and R. Kumar (Ed.), *Additive manufacturing for plastic recycling* (pp. 159–170). Boca Raton, FL: CRC Press.

Kumar, V., Singh, R. and Ahuja, I.S., 2022d. On rheological, thermal, mechanical, morpho-logical, and piezoelectric properties and one-way programming features of polyvinyli-dene fluoride–$CaCO_3$ composites. *Journal of Materials Engineering and Performance*, 31, pp. 4998–5012.

Lin, C., Liu, L., Liu, Y. and Leng, J., 2022. 4D printing of shape memory polybutylene suc-cinate/polylactic acid (PBS/PLA) and its potential applications. *Composite Structures*, 279, p. 114729.

Liu, X., Miao, J., Fan, Q., Zhang, W., Zuo, X., Tian, M., Zhu, S., Zhang, X. and Qu, L., 2022. Recent progress on smart fiber and textile based wearable strain sensors: Materials, fabrications, and applications. *Advanced Fiber Materials*. https://doi.org/10.1007/ s42765-021-00126-3.

Parratte, S. and Argenson, J.N., 2007. Validation and usefulness of a computer-assisted cup-positioning system in total hip arthroplasty: A prospective, randomized, controlled study. *Journal of Bone and Joint Surgery*, 89(3), pp. 494–499.

Ranjan, N., Kumar, R., Singh, R. and Kumar, V., 2021. On PVC-PP composite matrix for 4D applications: Flowability, mechanical, thermal, and morphological characterizations. *Journal of Thermoplastic Composite Materials*, p. 08927057211059754.

Rao, M.S. and Dave, B.C., 2002. Molecular design of organically-modified 'smart' sol-gel materials. *MRS Online Proceedings Library*, 726, p. 13. https://doi.org/10.1557/PROC -726-Q1.3.

Schmalzried, T.P., Guttmann, D., Grecula, M. and Amstutz, H.C., 1994. The relationship between the design, position, and articular wear of acetabular components inserted without cement and the development of pelvic osteolysis. *Journal of Bone and Joint Surgery*, 76(5), pp. 677–688.

Schwartz, M. (Ed.), 2008. *Smart Materials* (1st ed.). CRC Press. https://doi.org/10.1201 /9781420043730.

Seiler, M., 2006. Hyperbranched polymers: Phase behavior and new applications in the field of chemical engineering. *Fluid Phase Equilibria*, 241(1–2), pp. 155–174.

Seki, T., 2006. Photoresponsive self-assembly motions in polymer thin films. *Current Opinion in Solid State and Materials Science*, 10(5–6), pp. 241–248.

Sharma, R., Singh, R., Batish, A. and Ranjan, N., 2021. Investigations on chemical assisted mechanically blended 3D printed functional prototypes of PVDF-BaTiO3-Gr composite. Reference module in materials science and materials engineering. https://doi.org/10 .1016/B978-0-12-820352-1.00144-9.

Singh, R. and Kumar, R., 2020. Solid polymer waste materials for repairing of heritage composite structure: An additive manufacturing approach. In *Encyclopedia of Renewable and Sustainable Materials* (Vol. 4, pp. 557–562). Amsterdam, Netherlands: Elsevier.

Singh, R., Sharma, R. and Ranjan, N., 2017. Four-dimensional printing for clinical dentistry. Encyclopedia of smart materials. *Elsevier*, 1, pp. 329–355. https://doi.org/10.1016/B978 -0-12-803581-8.10167-5.

Song, J., Cheng, Q., Zhu, S. and Stevens, R.C., 2002. "Smart" materials for biosensing devices: Cell-mimicking supramolecular assemblies and colorimetric detection of pathogenic agents. *Biomedical Microdevices*, 4(3), pp. 213–221. https://doi.org/10.1023 /A:1016000530783.

Tomlinson, G.R. and Bullough, W.A. (Eds.), 1998. Smart materials and structures: Proceedings of the 4th European and 2nd MIMR Conference, Harrogate, UK, 6-8 July 1998 (1st ed.). CRC Press. https://doi.org/10.1201/9781482268560.

Zhang, Z., Demir, K.G. and Gu, G.X., 2019. Developments in 4D printing: A review on current smart materials, technologies, and applications. *International Journal of Smart and Nano Materials*, 10(3), pp. 205–224.

7 A Case Study on the Use of In-house Prepared Filaments for 4D Printing Applications in Orthopedics

Rupinder Singh and Abhishek Barwar

CONTENTS

7.1   INTRODUCTION

With technological advances in the field of additive manufacturing (AM) and medical imaging techniques, 3D models of the human body have been developed to rehearse complex surgical cases to eliminate any chance of error during actual operating conditions; whereas, in the case of veterinary patients these diagnostic techniques are not as common as in the field of human medicine (Harrysson et al., 2015).

However, in the past decade, veterinary medicine has also shown a rapid increase in specializations such as performing complex joint replacement, limb-sparing, radiation therapy with the use of advanced imaging techniques, as well as better surgical planning (Ohlerth et al., 2003). 3D modeling of complex bone-shapes has been proven effective in designing custom-based prostheses for patients with bone-loss following an accident (Liska et al., 2007). In the case of dogs, chondrodystrophy and stefal prostheses are the most commonly reported deformities which lead to angulation, abnormal growth of joints, length deficit, etc., and, to measure the degree of rotation or deficit of length, the use of 3D visualization software has been reported (Kwan et al., 2014). AM is used to manufacture the end product by utilizing the 3D CAD model as input by slicing the model into a number of cross-sectional layers (Rengier et al., 2010). 3D printing utilizes materials in the form of polymers, metal powder, ceramic, and bio-gels to fabricate patient-specific implants or scaffolds, and was found to be more economical than biomedical implants fabricated using other mechanical processes (Mulford et al., 2016).

4D (CT and MRI) imaging is a new scanning technique used to capture the images of a body part in multiple dimensions, including time, to determine the deformity more effectively (Kwong et al., 2015). The main purpose behind the up-grade of existing scanning techniques was to obtain images of body parts when they are in motion with great accuracy, and also to improve the quality of biomedical imaging (Schaverien et al., 2008; Nie et al., 2013). 4D images are proven to help design CAD models for 3D printing by converting the images into a specific format, and are also used for observing the shape changes of a 3D orthopedic model when it is given some sort of stimulus (Haleem and Javaid, 2019). Orthopedic implants developed by 3D printing techniques are already in use in the field of medicine and consume less fabrication time, but 4D printing is a trending method to develop similar kinds of implants (by using smart material) that can grow with time, depending on the age of the patient (Javaid and Haleem, 2019). The application of smart materials having 4D properties can help produce patient-specific orthopedic devices that are able to change their shape whenever some kind of stimulus (it may be in the form of heat, mechanical force, electrical, etc.) is applied to the material (Zhang et al., 2015; Bodaghi et al., 2019).

Shape-memory polymer (SMP) is the class of smart material (that can vary its shape or dimensions when some stimulus is provided) meant specifically for polymers other than shape-memory alloys (SMAs) (Leist et al., 2017). SMPs having key features such as biodegradability, non-toxicity, and biocompatibility are needed for biomedical applications such as drug delivery, bone-tissue engineering, bone-defect repair, self-tightening sutures, etc (Han et al., 2013; Tian et al., 2019). Among the naturally derived polyesters, PLA shows promising results (shape-memory effect (SME)) for a limited number of processing cycles (Lu et al., 2005), whereas when hydroxyapatite is reinforced in PLA-derived polymer it shows better shape recovery in the presence of a stimulus (Zheng et al., 2006). Some studies reported that the fabrication of foldable origami structures (by 3D printing using PLA-based feed-stock filaments) was usually programmed with some mechanical action and they were returned to their initial shape once glass-transition temperature occurred as the

SMPs were activated (Mehrpouya et al., 2020; Liu et al., 2018). The functional prototypes manufactured using PLA-HAP-CS–based composite feedstock filament will behave as osteo allografts for the surrounding osteoblast cells, which results in faster bone recovery (Ranjan et al., 2019). The literature survey reveals that the use of PLA and its copolymers has been reported for 4D printing applications, whereas the use of HAP and CS as the reinforcing materials was also practiced by some researchers for orthopedic applications; however, hitherto, little has been reported about the use of PLA-HAP-CS–based feedstock filament for 4D printing applications in the field of veterinary sciences.

To understand the gap in the literature, a bibliographic analysis has been performed by utilizing the past two decades' research data extracted from the web of science (WOS) knowledge base. Initially, the keywords "orthopedic applications", "3D printing", and "fused deposition modelling" were searched on the WOS platform and, as a result, the literature record of the past two decades has been obtained. To construct a networking diagram, the obtained data were processed through the VOSviewer software tool, the minimum occurrence of a term has been selected as 3, and based on that, 46 out of 876 total terms meet the threshold value. Table 7.1 highlights the relevance score calculated for each of the 46 threshold terms and due to the default setting in the software, the 60% most relevant terms (i.e., 28) were involved in the construction of the networking diagram (Figure 7.1).

Figure 7.1 outlines the linkage diagram based on the mutual research carried out for the terms "orthopedic applications", "FDM", and "3D printing" and as shown in Figure 7.1, three different clusters were formed representing the work reported in three different domains. Further, to investigate the research gap, the nodes "orthopedic" and "deposition modelling" were highlighted to check the linkage of these nodes with others and also the linkage strength as shown in Figure 7.1(a) and (b) respectively. It was found that the node "orthopedic" was connected with 3D printing and FDM but has been not directly connected with "porous scaffold" and PLA, which shows that little work was reported on the use of PLA-based material to develop scaffolds for orthopedic applications via 3D printing.

Similarly, Table 7.2 represents the terms used in the formation of the network diagram (Figure 7.2) using 1,030 total terms extracted from the WOS database for the past 20 years. Out of these 1,030 terms, 69 meet the threshold value by setting the minimum occurrence to 3, and 60% most relevant ones (i.e., 41) out of these 69 terms have contributed to the network diagram. The relevance score for each term has been calculated based on the appearance of the terms in the literature of the WOS database.

Figure 7.2 showcases the bibliographic diagram developed based on the keywords "4D printing", "scaffold", "biomedical", and "composite". The figure shows four different clusters formed representing the independent research carried out in four different areas. Similarly, on highlighting a particular node, the research gap has been ascertained. Figure 7.2(a) represents the shape-memory polymer that was reported for tissue-engineering applications but little has been reported on the use of the composition of different materials to carry out shape-memory effects. Similarly, Figure 7.2(b) highlights the connection of composition with biomedical applications

TABLE 7.1

Terms Used for the Formation of Networking Diagram and Relevance Score for Each Term

S. No.	Term	Occurrences	Relevance Score
1	3D printing	6	1.5035
2	Bone grafting	3	0.8051
3	Cell adhesion	3	0.4146
4	Compressive strength	3	0.755
5	Day	3	0.4315
6	Deposition modeling	7	0.5756
7	Dimensional printing	4	0.6267
8	Electron microscopy	5	1.4163
9	Fabrication	3	1.1169
10	Fused deposition modeling	3	0.7438
11	Implant	5	0.9741
12	Influence	3	0.6165
13	Morphology	4	0.7474
14	MPa	4	1.5133
15	Orthopedic	3	1.7859
16	PCL	3	0.4755
17	PLA	5	0.5164
18	Porosity	5	0.514
19	Porous scaffold	4	1.5133
20	Printing	3	2.9898
21	Process	4	1.4636
22	SEM	5	1.4163
23	Technology	6	1.4146
24	Tomography	6	0.4171
25	Use	5	1.9555
26	Value	5	0.6377
27	Vitro	5	0.3025
28	Work	4	0.3577

independently but not connected with smart materials which indicates that little work has been reported on the use of composite-based smart material for 4D printing.

7.2 METHODOLOGY

The proposed methodology for the preparation of feedstock filament for 4D printing applications:

- Identification of most-suited biocompatible materials (i.e., PLA, HAP, CS) for orthopedic applications.

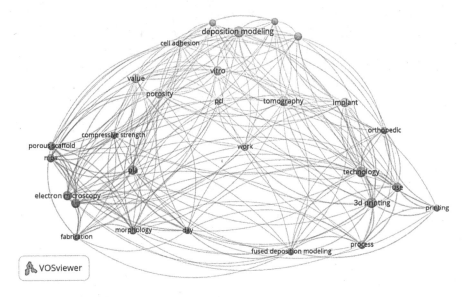

FIGURE 7.1 Bibliographic diagram based on the terms "FDM", "3D printing", and "orthopedic applications".

- Reinforcing of bioactive materials into PLA to make the orthopedic implants or scaffolds behave in almost the same way as natural bone.
- Analysis of melt-flow properties (viscosity, MFI) of the prepared composition by performing the MFI of the mixture prepared using a ball mill for 10Min as per ASTM 1238.
- Initially, extrusion of feedstock filaments on twin-screw extruder (TSE) was been performed, followed by crushing of the filaments carried out on a mechanical shredder for a fixed number of cycles (e.g., 3; 6; 9) for further processing onto SSE.
- To ascertain the effect of multiple extrusion of the material on its physical properties, the filaments were extruded through SSE having a standard die of 1.75mm.
- To analyze the mechanical strength of the material, the prepared filaments were tested on UTM for a strain rate of 30N/mm, as a result of which, certain mechanical properties of the material were obtained after the test.
- Surface characteristics of the fractured samples were obtained by performing the morphological analysis of the fractured cross-section.
- Electrical characteristics of the filament samples were performed by using an instrument i.e., a source measure unit, and as a result of the performed test, a relationship between voltage, resistance, and current was obtained.
- The shape-memory behavior of the PLA-based composite was analyzed by programming the feedstock filaments in hydro form and then observing the effect of the hydro-thermal stimulus on the prepared filaments by dipping the filament inside the water container at 37°C (Figure 7.3).

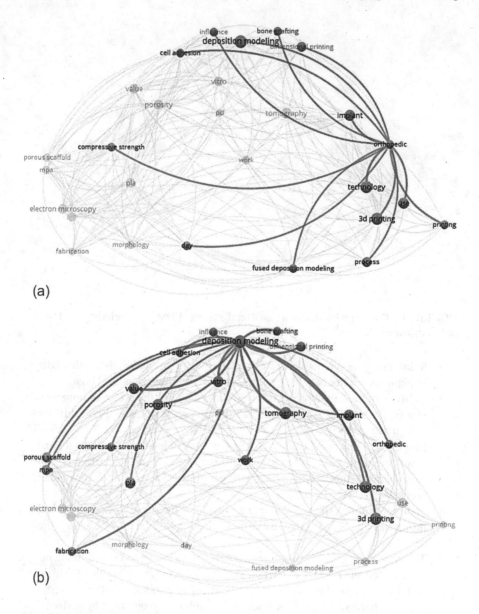

(a)

(b)

FIGURE 7.1(A) & (B) (a) Connections between different nodes upon highlighting orthopedic, (b) Gap analysis by highlighting deposition modeling.

7.3 MATERIAL SELECTION

To develop the feedstock filaments for 4D printing of orthopedic implants, or scaffolds, the material should be biocompatible as well as bioactive in nature. Hence, in this work, PLA, along with HAP and CS, has been used to prepare the composite

TABLE 7.2
Relevance Score for Each Term Based on the Terms "Biomedical", "4D Printing", "Composite", and "Scaffold"

S. No.	Term	Occurrences	Relevance Score
1	Advance	6	0.6154
2	Advantage	5	0.7068
3	Architecture	5	0.1688
4	Article	3	2.3551
5	Benefit	3	0.8025
6	Bio	3	0.3382
7	Biomedical engineering	4	0.3737
8	Bioprinting	4	1.1361
9	Category	3	0.5992
10	Cell	6	0.4868
11	Challenge	7	0.8189
12	Composition	3	1.083
13	Effort	4	1.3582
14	Evolution	3	0.548
15	Extrusion	5	0.5934
16	FDM	3	2.0962
17	Filament	5	1.4901
18	Future direction	3	1.8031
19	Last decade	3	0.9694
20	Manufacturing	13	0.2968
21	Mechanical property	6	0.417
22	Object	9	1.109
23	Paper	6	0.4737
24	Part	4	0.4688
25	Potential application	3	2.5236
26	Proliferation	3	0.2828
27	Property	8	1.557
28	Recent year	3	0.5003
29	Regenerative medicine	4	0.9168
30	Researcher	3	1.9952
31	Shape	8	0.387
32	Shape-memory effect	3	2.6601
33	Shape-memory polymer	4	1.7435
34	Smart material	8	0.6874
35	Stimulus	5	0.6052
36	Temperature	8	1.303
37	Tissue engineering	8	0.3367
38	Tissue-engineering application	3	0.5837
39	Variety	3	2.5528
40	Way	3	0.5682
41	Work	5	0.6883

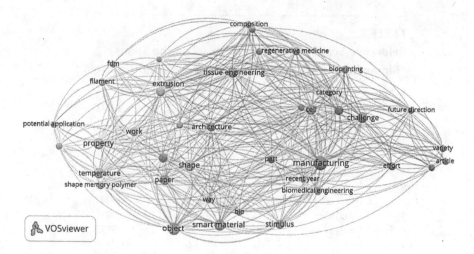

FIGURE 7.2 Networking diagram based upon the terms "composite", "biomedical", "scaffold", and "4D printing".

to develop a smart implant to continuously change the shape or volume when any kind of stimulus was provided to the material. HAP has been used broadly as a bone-repairing material specifically for orthopedic and dental implants (LeGeros and Legeros, 2008). Other than that, HAP possesses excellent biocompatibility with the surrounding tissues and supports the healing of the wounds, which makes it a suitable material for tissue-engineering applications (Lin and Chang, 2015). Since the end application of the smart material was to develop the patient-specific implant, henceforth CS, a polysaccharide generally derived from the shellfish, was used here to provide rich anti-micro bacterial properties along with an excellent wound-healing agent (Nurunnabi et al., 2017). To prepare the composite, different compositions were produced by varying the proportions of HAP and CS in PLA. Initially, the moisture content of the materials was removed by putting the materials (PLA granules at 60°C, but HAP and CS at 40°C) inside the heated oven for four hours separately and then properly mixed inside a ball mill for two hours (Ranjan et al., 2017). Once the materials are properly mixed, the flowability of the composite is ensured by performing MFI.

7.4   EXPERIMENTATION

7.4.1   FLOW CHARACTERISTICS

The flow behavior of the PLA-based composite was analyzed by performing the MFI as per ASTM D1238. According to this method, the material was inserted into the heated barrel and comes out in a molten state through a standard die under the action of applied load (2.160kg). To perform the MFI, three compositions were prepared i.e., PLA-HAP-CS (90-8-2, 91-7-2, and 92-6-2). The experiment was performed at 180°C by applying a load of 2.160kg. To minimize the error percentage contribution,

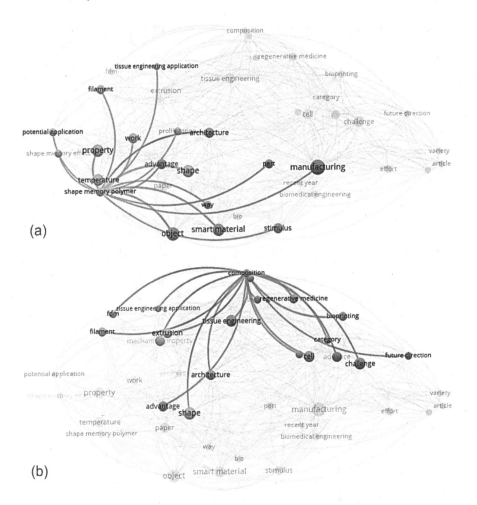

FIGURE 7.2(A) & (B) (a) Research gap identification by highlighting the term "shape-memory polymer", (b) gap analysis based upon the term "composition".

the test was performed for three sets of iterations for each composition and an average of them was considered.

7.4.2 PREPARATION OF FEEDSTOCK FILAMENTS

Once the flowability of the composite was established, the preparation stage of feedstock filament occurs in which the prepared composition was fed into the hopper of a twin-screw extruder (TSE) (for proper blending) and extruded at the preferred setting (T=180°C, N=85rpm, m=2.16kg) through a die of 1.75mm diameter. To analyze the effect of re-extrusion on the physical properties of the material, the prepared filaments were crushed using a mechanical shredder and then reprocessed through

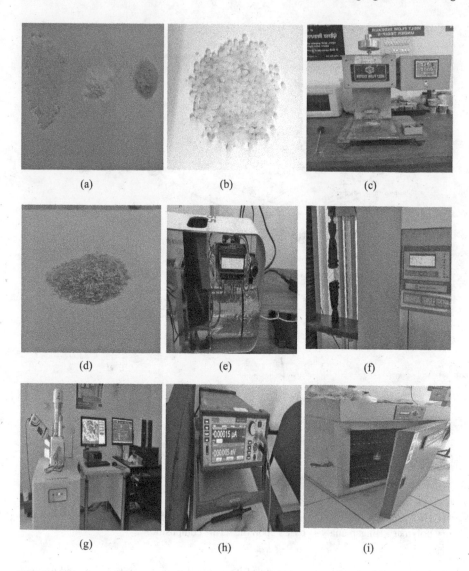

FIGURE 7.3 Process flow for the preparation of filaments.

an SSE by varying certain parameters (i.e., temperature, shredding cycles, and screw rpm), and a set of wires were prepared accordingly.

7.4.3 TENSILE TESTING

The set of extruded filaments (as per some input parameters of SSE) was then tested on a universal tensile testing setup having a maximum load capacity of 5000 N to determine the mechanical properties of the composite. The filaments were clamped in-between the fixtures and a continuous tensile load was applied on both ends of the filaments. The diameter of the wire was selected to be 1.75mm during the experiment and the mechanical properties were measured accordingly. The peak strain is the desired property required here merely to analyze the ability to recover shape when a stimulus is provided to the composite.

7.4.4 SCANNING ELECTRON MICROSCOPY (SEM)

To extract the surface characteristics, morphology was carried out by performing the SEM analysis at the cross-section of the fractured samples. The photomicrographs were taken at different magnification factors of the sample which showcases the highest value of strain. In addition to this, the porosity percentage of the sample (using SEM image at 100X) was carried out in metallurgical image analysis software (MIAS). Further, to determine the possible reason behind the fracture, the surface texture parameters – namely, amplitude distribution function (ADF), peak count (PC), rendered image, and average surface roughness (R_a) – were obtained by processing the micrograph in the Gwydion software as shown in Figure 7.4.

7.4.5 SHAPE-MEMORY BEHAVIOR

The shape-memory properties of the prepared feedstock filaments were analyzed by performing the specific test known as the aging effect; the filament samples were

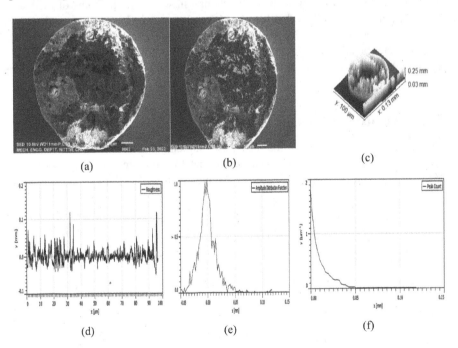

FIGURE 7.4 Surface texture analysis using the SEM photomicrograph at 100X.

weighed initially and then programmed by dipping the sample into the water-carrying container heated at 37°C for 24 hours. After 24 hours, the weight of the samples was measured and the corresponding change in volume of the filament sample was observed. The samples were provided the stimulus of open-environment conditions to see the effect on their dimensions. The process was repeated thrice to eliminate error.

7.4.6 ELECTRICAL PROPERTIES

To understand the electrical behavior of the prepared composite, the measurement of the V-I (voltage-current) and V-R (voltage-resistance) characteristics of the filament samples was carried out using a source measure unit (SMU). While performing the test, the samples were cut at equal length (i.e., 50mm) and held in-between the crocodile clamps of the electrodes. The graphs between V-I and V-R were developed by providing the input as sweep voltage for 10 seconds and the values of I and R were observed at 1.5V.

7.5 RESULTS AND DISCUSSION

7.5.1 MELT-FLOW BEHAVIOR

The flowability analysis of the composite material (PLA-HAP-CS) was carried out based on the MFI results for different sets of compositions. Figure 7.5 shows the trend of MFI (in g/10min) with the change in weight proportions of PLA and HAP. The measured MFI value for the compositions was 7.378, 9.916, and 10.268 respectively for 90-8-2, 91-7-2, and 92-6-2. The trend indicates that the MFI of the prepared composition increases with a decrease in the weight proportion of HAP, keeping the constant weight of CS. The reason behind such MFI behavior may be the higher density of HAP in comparison to PLA (Liu et al., 2019).

7.5.2 MECHANICAL CHARACTERISTICS

The mechanical properties of the feedstock filaments drawn through the combination of both TSE and SSE were analyzed by performing the UTM test at the preferred strain rate of 30N/mm. Figure 7.6 indicates that the filament exhibits great

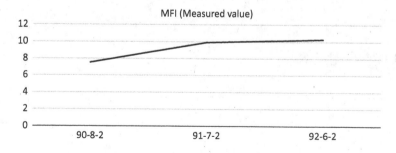

FIGURE 7.5   MFI trend of PLA-HAP-CS for different compositions.

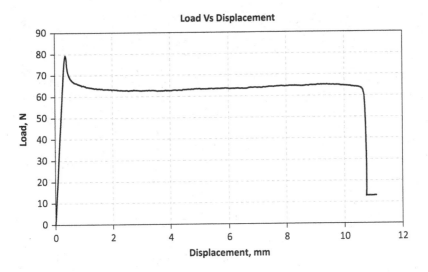

Load Vs Displacement

FIGURE 7.6 Load v/s deformation curve of the tested sample on UTM.

elasticity as the observed value for peak load is 79.55N and the elongation at break was noted to be 65.867%. Since the filament was drawn for 4D printing applications the peak strain may be the noticeable property and the strain percentage maximum load was found to be 2.293.

7.5.3 SURFACE CHARACTERISTICS

Morphology of the fractured filament samples has been established by capturing the photomicrographs at 100X, and the surface texture of the fractured site was analyzed by measuring the roughness parameters in the Gwyddion software tool at a cut-off length of 0.0156um. The obtained value of average roughness (R_a=13.86um) indicates the uniform mixing of materials, whereas the ADF indicates that the curve has followed a normal distribution curve. (i.e., uniformly distributed). A 3D rendered image of the cross-section represents lesser peaks and valleys; as shown in the PC curve, the maximum value of peak occurred at 0.25mm. The porosity percentage was observed to be 3.83%, which may be the reason behind the higher value of peak strength.

7.5.4 V-I AND V-R CHARACTERISTICS

To understand the electrical behavior of the prepared feedstock filaments, the V-I and V-R characteristic curves were plotted before and after having been given the stimulus using SMU interlinked with Kickstart software. Figure 7.7 shows that the value of resistance corresponding to 1.5V was 118Ω, whereas after providing the stimulus, the value of resistance was limited to 55Ω only. The decrease in resistance may be due to less porosity of the material and also because of the stimulus in hydro form.

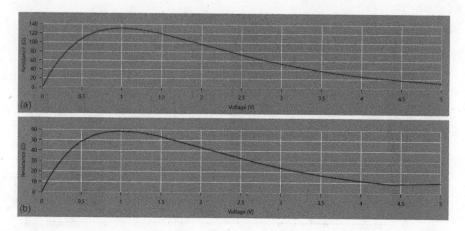

FIGURE 7.7   V-I and V-R characteristic curves of filaments before and after the stimulus effect.

7.5.5 Shape-Memory Effect

To identify the shape-memory effect, initially the filament was weighed at 0.04g, and after 24 hours the weight of the samples was measured as 0.0412g. During hydro-thermal programming, the filament samples were deformed from 20.08mm to 20.16mm longitudinally, whereas the diameter also increased from 1.43 to 1.46mm. Moving ahead, stimulus in the form of open-environment conditions was provided to the samples, and shape recovery was observed as: final length, 20.10mm and final diameter, 1.44mm. For typical suture applications in the case of veterinary patients, this kind of shape recovery is desired (Liska et al., 2007).

7.6 SUMMARY

- The melt-flow behavior for the prepared composition provides satisfactory results while showing a continuous flow for all the cases, which indicates that the inclusion of HAP in the composite should be limited to 7–8% only for better extrusion of feedstock filaments as well as to prepare the implants with the high desired strength.
- Filament samples extruded at T=170°C, screw rpm (N)=5, and shredding parameter=6 show maximum value of peak strain i.e., 2.293, and elongation at break was reported as 65.86% which was suitable for the preparation of scaffolds.
- Morphology of the fractured sample suggests that the peaks were ranging from 0.03mm to 0.25mm (i.e., low average roughness) which represents the better blending and mixing of materials with each other. A lower value of R_a and porosity percentage was suitable for developing high-strength 3D printed orthopedic implants.

- The electrical characteristics show that the electric resistance of the material decrease after providing the stimulus, which indicates that the dielectric constant of the material will increase, which represents the reduction in radiation efficiency (Singh et al., 2022).
- The observations for the shape-memory test were that the initially programmed filaments were able to gain their shapes after providing the stimulus in hydro-thermal form. The shape recovery was observed to be 99.11%, which was desired for the development of smart orthopedic implants.

REFERENCES

Bodaghi, M., Noroozi, R., Zolfagharian, A., Fotouhi, M. and Norouzi, S., 2019. 4D printing self-morphing structures. *Materials*, 12(8), p. 1353.

Haleem, A. and Javaid, M., 2019. Expected role of four-dimensional (4D) CT and four-dimensional (4D) MRI for the manufacturing of smart orthopaedics implants using 4D printing. *Journal of Clinical Orthopaedics and Trauma*, 10, pp. S234–S235.

Han, J., Fei, G., Li, G. and Xia, H., 2013. High-intensity focused ultrasound triggered shape memory and drug release from biodegradable polyurethane. *Macromolecular Chemistry and Physics*, 214(11), pp. 1195–1203.

Harrysson, O.L., Marcellin-Little, D.J. and Horn, T.J., 2015. Applications of metal additive manufacturing in veterinary orthopedic surgery. *JOM*, 67(3), pp. 647–654.

Javaid, M. and Haleem, A., 2019. 4D printing applications in medical field: A brief review. *Clinical Epidemiology and Global Health*, 7(3), pp. 317–321.

Kwan, T.W., Marcellin-Little, D.J. and Harrysson, O.L., 2014. Correction of biapical radial deformities by use of bi-level hinged circular external fixation and distraction osteogenesis in 13 dogs. *Veterinary Surgery*, 43(3), pp. 316–329.

Kwong, Y., Mel, A.O., Wheeler, G. and Troupis, J.M., 2015. Four-dimensional computed tomography (4DCT): A review of the current status and applications. *Journal of Medical Imaging and Radiation Oncology*, 59(5), pp. 545–554.

LeGeros, R.Z. and LeGeros, J.P., 2008. Hydroxyapatite. In T. Kokubo (Ed.), *Bioceramics and their Clinical Applications* (pp. 367–394). Sawston: Woodhead Publishing Series in Biomaterials.

Leist, S.K., Gao, D., Chiou, R. and Zhou, J., 2017. Investigating the shape memory properties of 4D printed polylactic acid (PLA) and the concept of 4D printing onto nylon fabrics for the creation of smart textiles. *Virtual and Physical Prototyping*, 12(4), pp. 290–300.

Lin, K. and Chang, J., 2015. Structure and properties of hydroxyapatite for biomedical applications. In T. Kokubo (Ed.), *Hydroxyapatite (HAp) for Biomedical Applications* (pp. 3–19). Sawston: Woodhead Publishing Series in Biomaterials.

Liska, W.D., Marcellin-Little, D.J., Eskelinen, E.V., Sidebotham, C.G., Harrysson, O.L. and Hielm-Björkman, A.K., 2007. Custom total knee replacement in a dog with femoral condylar bone loss. *Veterinary Surgery*, 36(4), pp. 293–301.

Liu, S., Li, Y., Sun, H., Zhang, S., Zeng, X., Zong, P., Wan, Y. and Zuo, G., 2019. Preparation and characterisation of a lamellar hydroxyapatite/polylactic acid composite. *Plastics, Rubber, and Composites*, 48(2), pp. 66–73.

Liu, Y., Zhang, W., Zhang, F., Lan, X., Leng, J., Liu, S., Jia X, Cotton C, Sun B and Gu B and Chou, T.W., 2018. Shape memory behavior and recovery force of 4D printed laminated Miura-origami structures subjected to compressive loading. *Composites Part B: Engineering*, 15(153), pp. 233–242.

Lu, X., Cai, W. and Zhao, L.C., 2005. Study on the shape memory behavior of poly (L-lactide). *Materials Science Forum*, 475, pp. 2399–2402.

Mehrpouya, M., Azizi, A., Janbaz, S. and Gisario, A., 2020. Investigation on the functionality of thermoresponsive origami structures. *Advanced Engineering Materials*, 22(8), p. 2000296.

Mulford, J.S., Babazadeh, S. and Mackay, N., 2016. Three-dimensional printing in orthopaedic surgery: Review of current and future applications. *ANZ Journal of Surgery*, 86(9), pp. 648–653.

Nie, J.Y., Lu, L.J., Gong, X., Li, Q. and Nie, J.J., 2013. Delineating the vascular territory (perform some) of a perforator in the lower extremity of the rabbit with four-dimensional computed tomographic angiography. *Plastic and Reconstructive Surgery*, 131(3), pp. 565–571.

Nurunnabi, M., Revuri, V., Huh, K.M. and Lee, Y.K., 2017. Polysaccharide-based Nano/micro formulation: An effective and versatile oral drug delivery system. In E. Andronescu and A.M. Grumezescu (Eds.), *Nanostructures for Oral Medicine: Micro and Nano Technologies* (pp. 409–433). Amsterdam, Netherlands: Elsevier. https://doi.org/10.1016/B978-0-323-47720-8.00015-8.

Ohlerth, S., Busato, A., Rauch, M., Weber, U. and Lang, J., 2003. Comparison of three distraction methods and conventional radiography for early diagnosis of canine hip dysplasia. *Journal of Small Animal Practice*, 44(12), pp. 524–529.

Ranjan, N.I., Singh, R.U., Ahuja, I.P. and Singh, J.A., 2017. A framework for development of biocompatible feedstock filament of polymers by reinforcement of fillers for FDM. *International Journal of Materials Science and Engineering*, 8(2), pp. 185–189.

Ranjan, N., Singh, R., Ahuja, I.P. and Singh, J., 2019. Fabrication of PLA-HAp-CS based biocompatible and biodegradable feedstock filament using twin-screw extrusion. In Dr. B. AlMangour (Eds.), *Additive Manufacturing of Emerging Materials* (pp. 325–345). Cham: Springer.

Rengier, F., Mehndiratta, A., Von Tengg-Kobligk, H., Zechmann, C.M., Unterhinninghofen, R., Kauczor, H.U. and Giesel, F.L., 2010. 3D printing based on imaging data: Review of medical applications. *International Journal of Computer-Assisted Radiology and Surgery*, 5(4), pp. 335–341.

Schaverien, M., Saint-Cyr, M., Arbique, G., Hatef, D., Brown, S.A. and Rohrich, R.J., 2008. Three-and four-dimensional computed tomographic angiography and venography of the anterolateral thigh perforator flap. *Plastic and Reconstructive Surgery*, 121(5), pp. 1685–1696.

Singh, R., Barwar, A. and Kumar, A., 2022. Investigations on primary and secondary recycling of PLA and its composite for biomedical and sensing applications. *Journal of the Institution of Engineers (India): Series C*, 11, pp. 1–6.

Tian, G., Zhu, G., Xu, S. and Ren, T., 2019. A novel shape memory poly (ε-caprolactone)/hydroxyapatite nanoparticle networks for potential biomedical applications. *Journal of Solid State Chemistry*, 1(272), pp. 78–86.

Zhang, Q., Yan, D., Zhang, K. and Hu, G., 2015. Pattern transformation of heat-shrinkable polymer by three-dimensional (3D) printing technique. *Scientific Reports*, 5(1), pp. 1–6.

Zheng, X., Zhou, S., Li, X. and Weng, J., 2006. Shape memory properties of poly (D, L-lactide)/hydroxyapatite composites. *Biomaterials*, 27(24), pp. 4288–4295.

8 A Case Study of 4D-Imaging-Assisted 4D Printing for Clinical Dentistry for Canines

Smruti Ranjan Pradhan, Minhaz Husain,
Rupinder Singh, and Sukhwant Singh Banwait

CONTENTS

8.1 INTRODUCTION

The engineering processes are divided into two categories: forward and reverse engineering. Forward engineering is the established process where logical designs with high-level abstractions are physically implemented in a well-planned system to develop a product. This may or may not include a detailed drawing with a list of materials and raw data processing for developing a new physical product. The desire to accelerate advanced intelligence and to have interdisciplinary access to new complexities has led to the establishment of modern additive manufacturing (AM) technology that uses digital blueprints such as computer-aided design (CAD) models. On the other hand, reverse engineering is the duplication of an existing product that includes the systematic joining of point clouds for the development of a meaningful virtual model through 3D scanning and CAD modeling (Raja and Fernandes, 2007). 3D printing initiated research into applications ranging from biomedical to electronics and, most prominently, in biomimetics and smart materials for the advantages of convenience and adept object production, thanks to the effectiveness of material usability, surface resolution, and finely tuned design.

The static and inanimate existence of the printed object, including the anisotropic behavioral patterns of the technology, acted as a barrier in printing technology, which was eliminated by 4D printing, which added a temporal dimension to 3D concepts and offered substance to the design by using a stimulus to trigger

DOI: 10.1201/9781003205531-8

transfiguration into smart materials. On acquaintance with specific additional stimuli, such as calefaction, moisture, light, active springs, electromagnetic radiations, and pH attributed to martensitic transformation (such as intrinsic elasticity), smart materials consisting of hydrogels, ceramics, metals, alloys, and polymers tend toward origami. However, polymers are among the most promising materials for 4D printing due to their high rigidity, dominant recoverable strain (up to 800%), ability to trigger shape recoverability (in bending, 93% and tensile, 87%), and ease of fabrication into tailor-made products, with some exhibiting biodegradability and biocompatibility. This chapter examines recent advances in 4D printing, focusing on smart polymers and cognate stimuli response, material compatibility with 3D printers, applications, and 4D printing of SMP trends (Subash and Kandasubramanian, 2020; Aber et al., 2010). The different steps associated with 4D printing are given in Figure 8.1.

3D printing has been touted as a game-changing technology and has already piqued the medical community's curiosity. Prototypes duplicated for broken components and even complete organs can be made using patient-specific designs and 3D models. For example, the bespoke Talus spacer could be an excellent alternative in trauma cases where the surrounding joint has significant cartilage. The 3D talus was created using bilateral ankle CT as a design input. On the damaged talus, the healthy side talus was mirrored and registered. Before operation planning, design ideas are carefully taken by considering the talus size differences caused by soft-tissue balancing (upsize, downsize, natural).

Photogrammetry is the art of capturing, scientifically measuring, and implementing new technology for interpreting photographic images and patterns of recorded radiant electromagnetic energy and other phenomena to gain reliable information about physical objects and the environment. Photogrammetry predates photography by almost a century. Since its inception around 150 years ago, photogrammetry has progressed from a purely analog, optical-mechanical technique to analytical methods based on the computer-aided solution of mathematical algorithms, and finally to digital or softcopy photogrammetry based on digital imagery and computer vision, which is devoid of any optomechanical hardware. Photogrammetry accurately measures three-dimensional objects and terrain features from two-dimensional photos. Coordinate measurement, distance, height, area, and volume calculation, topographic map preparation, and the creation of digital elevation models and orthophotographs are all typical applications of this. Photogrammetry is a valuable technology that can

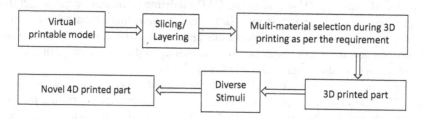

FIGURE 8.1 Steps associated with 4D printing.

be implemented in implant dentistry to find the accuracy of tool in clinical applications, aiding the coordinated transfer of implants (Hussein, M.O., 2021).

The number of studies on 4D, 5D, and 6D printing has recently increased. This study examines and analyses existing 4D printing uses, benefits, limitations, and challenges. The food-printing industry also studies the concepts, actual applications, and possible applications of the most recent additive manufacturing technologies (5D and 6D printing). Currently, 4D food-print implementations have primarily concentrated on improving the color, shape, flavor, and nutritional aspects of 3D printed-food items. Furthermore, 5D and 6D printing have the potential to manufacture highly complex structures with greater strength and less material than 3D and 4D printing. These new technologies are projected to lead to substantial future advancements in various industries, including manufacturing high-quality food products that are currently impossible to make with current processing technology. The goal of this research is to identify the industrial potential of 4D printing and the possibilities for further innovation using 5D and 6D printing (Ghazal et al., 2022). The different attributes affecting 4D printing are given in Figure 8.2.

Multiple material printing corresponding to a particular layer during precise 3D printing of a model leads to a controlled heterogeneous microstructure. The 4D printing principle is used in the design and manufacture of active origami, in which a flat sheet folds into a complex 3D component autonomously. Here the shape-memory polymer fibers are precisely printed in an elastomeric matrix of active composites that can be used as intelligent functional hinges to enable origami folding patterns.

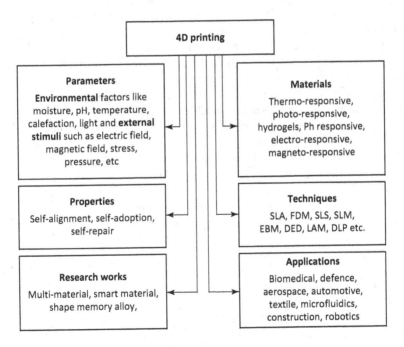

FIGURE 8.2 Different attributes of 4D printing.

The theoretical model aids in selecting design factors such as fiber-size, hinge-length, and strain and temperature programming, which are essential to building numerous active origami components from flat polymer sheets, including a box, a pyramid, and two origami planes, using the model (Ge et al. 2014). High-fidelity finite element simulations were used to precisely anticipate the nonlinear deformation of printed structures to determine crucial design parameters such as local deformation, shape persistence, and recovery ratio (Akbari et al., 2018).

3D printing has already aided the dental industry by making custom-specific 3D dental crowns. Due to digitization, dentists may now produce bridges, crowns, orthodontic appliances, and die-stone models quickly and correctly using various design tools and scanning technology. 4D printing is a new technological advancement that can revolutionize restorative dentistry. 4D printed functional products are expected to replace 3D printed products shortly. The notion of 4D printing was launched in 2012 and sparked interest in planning, procedures, and material selections. A 4D printing method allows a printed model/product to alter shape and function in response to environmental conditions such as heat, water, light, and electricity over time. The special shape-memory alloys can be used to adjust the deformation as per the functional requirements concerning time. So, the 3D printing of dental prostheses and orthoses can be done in such a way that an external stimulus can enhance the shape-change of a particular product. It is considered a revolutionary 4D printed product with the expense of smart material. So, partial tooth loss can be treated with this technique as it requires further growth to rebuild the tooth structure. However, commercially, this think-tank technique is not feasible at present. The jaw-tracking integration dentistry technique has been used as a new low-cost workflow for integrating mandible kinematics into a static virtual patient. Here the data from computed tomography is segmented and combined with intraoral surface scans and a target tracking video that mimics mandible movements. An open-source virtual reality software tool was used to generate a 4D dynamic virtual patient. All patient-specific parameters can be exported to individualize an analog or virtual articulator (Zambrana et al., 2022; Khorsandi et al., 2021).

A bibliographic study has been adopted using VOSviewer software to find the research gap. This web of science database (past two decades) was implemented with the keywords 4D imaging and 4D printing. A total of 114 results were found. These results were extracted in a .text file and analyzed by VOSviewer software (Table 8.1 and Figure 8.3 (a)). In Figure 8.3, when a node is highlighted, it shows the relationship of the particular node with the other points (Figure 8.3 (b, c, d, e, f, g, h)). This also shows a strong or weak nodal path for better literature analysis.

8.2   MATERIAL AND METHODS FOR 4D PRINTING IN DENTISTRY

Vinyl polymer is made by free radical polymerization from vinyl monomers. Though it is biocompatible, it is not used for implant applications due to its poor biodegradable characteristics, although it is a promising material for the dental industry. 4D properties, such as variation of molecular weight, are enhanced in this material by implementing control radical polymerization. These polymers are extensively used

TABLE 8.1
Relevance Score of Various Terms Used in Extracting
Bibliographic-Based Network Diagram

Id	Term	Occurrences	Relevance Score
1	3D geometry	3	1.3005
2	3D model	4	0.8703
3	3D printer	4	0.5206
4	3D printing technology	3	0.6353
5	4D bioprinting	3	1.6925
6	4D flow	7	0.9685
7	4D imaging	4	0.7476
8	Accuracy	7	0.6906
9	Adaptability	4	0.6999
10	Advance	8	0.9012
11	Algorithm	5	0.8356
12	Alignment	5	1.4726
13	Amplitude	3	0.9717
14	Anatomy	7	0.4622
15	Aneurysm	8	0.9434
16	Angular information	3	1.3829
17	Architecture	13	1.029
18	Article	4	1.4983
19	Author	3	0.8375
20	Behavior	3	1.7239
21	Bio ink	5	1.6893
22	Biomedicine	3	1.2302
23	Bioprinting	6	1.4957
24	Case	8	0.6664
25	Cell	13	0.9368
26	Cerebral aneurysm	3	0.8773
27	CFD	4	1.0655
28	Change	14	0.5405
29	Coating	4	0.7467
30	Color	7	1.7354
31	Complexity	6	0.4891
32	Composition	7	0.8532
33	Computational fluid dynamic	4	1.0188
34	Computed tomography	6	0.5406
35	Construct	9	1.439
36	Curvature	3	0.9363
37	Custom	3	0.5079
38	Deformation	7	0.856
39	Degrees c	7	1.1322
40	Densification	3	0.7395

(*Continued*)

TABLE 8.1 (CONTINUED)
Relevance Score of Various Terms Used in Extracting
Bibliographic-Based Network Diagram

Id	Term	Occurrences	Relevance Score
41	Deposition	3	0.6717
42	Deposition modeling	4	0.3729
43	Difference	12	0.4797
44	Differential scanning calorimetry	3	0.9581
45	Digital light processing	4	1.3129
46	End	4	0.4504
47	Evaluation	9	0.3736
48	Example	4	1.5053
49	Experimental result	3	0.7949
50	Fabrication	11	0.9296
51	Fdm	4	0.4874
52	Feasibility	4	0.8394
53	Filament	6	1.2978
54	Flow	20	0.7146
55	Flow MRI	5	1.0865
56	Flow pattern	8	0.9897
57	Formation	10	0.9815
58	Function	9	0.8688
59	Generation	5	1.0126
60	Good agreement	5	0.4388
61	Hemodynamic	7	1.0019
62	Hemodynamics	4	1.0171
63	High resolution	5	0.5
64	Hydrogel	8	1.0349
65	Impact	7	0.3132
66	Index	5	0.5617
67	Inspiration	3	1.0451
68	Intracranial aneurysm	4	1.2397
69	Lack	3	0.5565
70	Last decade	3	0.8494
71	Lce	3	1.832
72	Lces	3	1.832
73	Length scale	3	0.959
74	Light	6	1.1672
75	Location	4	0.7556
76	Magnetic resonance imaging	14	0.5655
77	Maximum	3	0.9067
78	Mean	4	0.5831
79	Mean difference	3	0.9178

(Continued)

TABLE 8.1 (CONTINUED)
Relevance Score of Various Terms Used in Extracting Bibliographic-Based Network Diagram

Id	Term	Occurrences	Relevance Score
80	Measurement	19	0.3107
81	Microstructure	6	0.8969
82	MRI	16	0.614
83	Nanostructure	3	4.3915
84	Nanostructured surface	3	4.7064
85	Need	4	0.553
86	Pathophysiology	3	0.9989
87	Patient	14	0.4814
88	Patient specific	3	0.8017
89	Peak	3	1.0674
90	Perspective	6	0.8459
91	Phantom	15	0.6425
92	Phase	5	0.4456
93	Phase separation	3	2.0336
94	Photoinitiator	3	1.3656
95	PLA	6	1.1264
96	Poly	4	1.175
97	Polylactic acid	6	0.8426
98	Polymer	7	1.0903
99	Position	7	0.5819
100	Post	3	0.6252
101	Potential application	4	1.3382
102	Print	5	1.3439
103	Printed model	6	0.7656
104	Printed structure	3	1.2764
105	Progress	3	1.0349
106	Quantification	7	0.573
107	Radiotherapy	4	0.794
108	Realistic representation	3	0.7782
109	Relation	4	1.0159
110	Reliability	3	0.4974
111	Replicas	3	0.8057
112	Reproducibility	3	0.6267
113	Respiratory motion	3	1.0357
114	Response	10	0.841
115	Reversible shape change	3	1.7985
116	Review	7	0.5812
117	Role	9	0.4482
118	Scaffold	10	0.9093
119	Scan	6	0.6274

(Continued)

TABLE 8.1 (CONTINUED)
Relevance Score of Various Terms Used in Extracting
Bibliographic-Based Network Diagram

Id	Term	Occurrences	Relevance Score
120	Set	7	0.6989
121	Shape-memory polymer	7	1.2846
122	Shear	3	0.6767
123	Smart material	5	0.9277
124	SMP	3	2.0306
125	Soft robotic	4	1.5863
126	Specimen	3	2.0462
127	Strategy	10	1.0109
128	Stress	4	0.7891
129	Subject	4	0.8186
130	Temperature	12	0.8649
131	Theory	4	0.8601
132	Tissue engineering	8	1.1703
133	Top	3	3.6024
134	Training	4	0.6566
135	Transition	4	0.7386
136	Treatment	8	0.3311
137	Validation	5	0.6279
138	Variety	4	1.333
139	Velocity	9	1.0336
140	Vitro	6	0.532
141	Vitro model	3	0.9615
142	Vivo	4	0.8174
143	Vorticity	3	1.0283

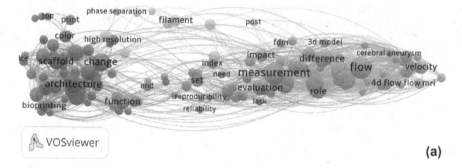

(a)

FIGURE 8.3   (a): The cluster obtained from VOSviewer software.

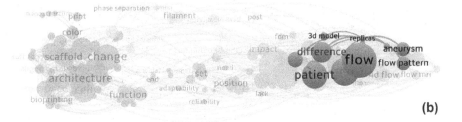

FIGURE 8.3   (b): Relationship of replicas with other areas.

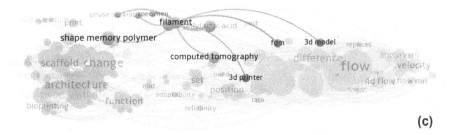

FIGURE 8.3   (c): Relationship of filament with other areas.

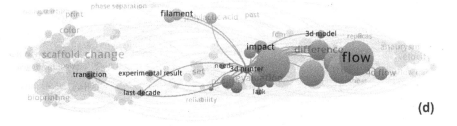

FIGURE 8.3   (d): Relationship of a 3D printer with other areas.

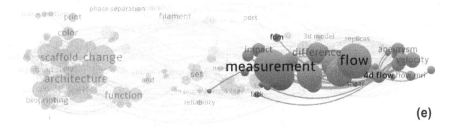

FIGURE 8.3   (e): Relationship of 4D flow with other areas.

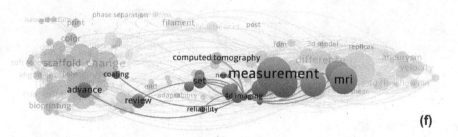

FIGURE 8.3   (f): Relationship of 4D imaging with other areas.

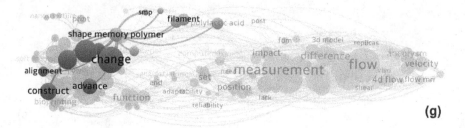

FIGURE 8.3   (g): Relationship of shape-memory polymers with other areas.

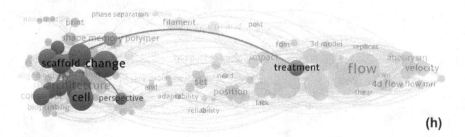

FIGURE 8.3   (h): Relation between scaffolds with other areas.

in SLS and SLA (Pradhan et al., 2021b; Stansbury and Idacavage, 2016; Shirazi et al., 2015). Due to its poor surface and mechanical properties, it is blended with polyetheretherketone, Al_2O_3, and SiO_2. Also, the further addition of TiO_2 enhances the antibacterial properties. Polycaprolactone, polycarbonate, polylactic acid, and acrylonitrile butadiene styrene are also promising polymers used in fused filament fabrication-based 3D printing for dental applications.

Metals are widely used in biocompatible device fabrication, mainly where corrosion and wear resistance are required. When choosing metal/alloy for biomedical purposes, mechanical characteristics and biocompatibility are also crucial considerations. A metallic material's biocompatibility refers to its ability to execute its intended function without causing unwanted local or systemic impacts on the tissues around it. Even though many different types of metallic materials exist, only a few are biologically compatible with the living body and can be employed for long-term applications. Stainless steel (316L, 17 4 PH, 302 SS, Vanadium steel, etc.) has been widely implemented as implants. The presence of Mo, and Cr yields corrosion resistance. Commercial pure titanium and Ti6Al4V are the widely used Ti-based medical-grade alloys. Wrought CoNiCrMo alloy (F562), wrought CoCrWNi alloy (F90), Cast CoCrMo alloy (F75), and wrought CoNiCrMoWFe (F563) alloy are four types of CoCr-based alloys available for biomedical applications. Cobalt chromium molybdenum (CoCrMo) alloys are of particular interest among CoCr alloys because of their superior corrosion and wear resistance, high tensile and yield strength, and biocompatibility.

Biocompatible ceramics have excellent properties such as wear resistance, shear bond strength, and better aesthetics than their metallic counterpart. Alumina and Zirconia are widely adopted ceramics in dental practices such as implant, abutment, endodontic posts, and crown-making (Pradhan et al., 2021c; Li et al., 2020). Various approaches for improving osteoblast adhesion, differentiation, and osseointegration of bone-implant filler were applied to further surface-treat ceramics. Surface roughening, surface coating with active components to turn a bio-inert surface into a bio-interactive surface, and lowering surface contaminants to improve surface hydrophilicity are the three major surface treatment strategies used (Pradhan et al., 2022; Hisbergues et al., 2009). Some of these procedures include surface modification with acid etching, hydrogen peroxide treatment, oxygen plasma, and UV irradiation. Ceramic-based biomaterials have been shown to inhibit inflammatory activity, plaque build-up, and bacterial colonization by altering fibroblast adhesion and proliferation (Pradhan et al., 2021a; Vickers, 2017).

3D printing is combined with the use of responsive materials, which adapt their properties or shape in response to chemical, electrical, or thermal stimuli (Pradhan et al., 2020; Bruni, 2019). Smart materials come in two varieties: shape-memory and shape-changing. To manufacture shape-memory materials, alloys, polymers, and ceramics can be employed. Each material has advantages and disadvantages, depending on its intended purpose. In dentistry, shape-memory polymers are used in endodontics, orthodontics, oral surgery, prosthodontics, and implantology. These systems should use sensitive materials to build a 3D-printed object that responds to external or internal stimuli (Choong et al., 2017; Sun et al., 2020). Magnetic nanoscale components such as Fe, Co, and Ni, together with a small amount of Cu and Zn, are often incorporated into raw materials to produce magnetically sensitive materials. These nanoparticles can be printed on-site (embedded) or mixed with predetermined ingredients (Zare et al., 2019).

Electrically sensitive materials are made from inherently conductive polymers such as polyacetylene, polyaniline, polypyrrole, and polythiophene, as well as their derivatives/copolymers. This could also be done with metal nanoparticles and conductive carbon-based nanostructures (Zare et al., 2013). Photosensitive metal nanostructures, as well as light-conducting materials or compounds containing azobenzene, stilbene, Spiro pyran, fulgide, or diarylethene, are used to make light-responsive materials (such as gold, platinum, and TiO_2) (Cui et al., 2019; Hingorani et al., 2019). Ultrasonic-sensitive materials are made of polymers whose bonds are cleaved when exposed to high ultrasound intensity. Biodegradable (e.g., polyglycolide and poly-lactides) and non-biodegradable polymers (collagen, gelatin, soybean oil epoxidized acrylate, pluronic, and polyether urethane) are common thermo-responsive materials used in 4D printing (Makvandi et al., 2020; Manouras and Vamvakaki, 2017). Due to the presence of functional groups such as hydroxyl (OH), carboxylic (COOH), sulfonic acid (SO_3H), and amine (NH_2) groups in the polymer chain, pH-sensitive materials swell or collapse depending on the surrounding pH. Moisture-sensitive materials (e.g., hydrogels) are similar to pH-responsive systems because they feature a hydrophilic functional group. Because of their hydrophilicity, the systems swell to a larger volume than before (Makvandi, P. et al., 2019).

Another type of material is one that reacts to biological stimuli, such as glucose and enzymes. Innovative materials that release insulin in reaction to blood-sugar levels, for example, could be used to control blood-glucose levels. Self-adaptability, shape memory, self-sensing, self-repair, self-responsiveness, and multi-functionality are all features of smart materials. Shape-memory materials, which restore their original shape after a stimulus, and shape-changing materials, which preserve their original shape but undergo a morphological change in response to a stimulus, are the two basic types of smart materials (Zhou et al., 2020). In 2012, researchers began experiment-ing with 4D printing in the dental field. Even though the technique isn't currently commercially accessible, it represents a significant advancement in AM capacity. 4D printed dental implants, for example, can change shape in response to changes in oral temperature and humidity, as well as diabetic circumstances. These implants have features that are similar to those seen in natural teeth (Javaid and Haleem, 2019).

The biomechanical qualities of different materials are associated with restorative dentistry color stability, strength, longevity, adhesion, and failure. When it comes to rebuilding the missing tooth structure, the oral environment presents difficul-ties due to its dynamic nature and functional and balancing pressures. Dimensional changes at the margins significantly cause restorative material failure, resulting in filling instability or total loss. 4D printed materials that perform constant self-fold-ing changes can move toward the edges, preventing microleakage and overhangs at the edges. 4D printing materials can move in specific directions that have been programmed before manufacture. By adjusting the motion path, these materials in restorative dentistry can reduce the need for dental adhesives (etching and bonding system) by relying on mechanical rather than chemical retention. Also, to ensure optimal adaptability, these restorative materials can be controlled to travel down-ward toward the tooth's fitting surface.

Furthermore, 4D printed fillings can be employed in inaccessible parts of the oral cavity where existing restorative materials are difficult to manipulate and maintain. Removable and fixed prosthodontic applications can also benefit from 4D printing. The method can create materials with qualities similar to those of genuine hard and soft tissues. The denture base can be made of structures with the same elasticity and temperature properties as periodontal ligaments or the overlying mucosa. In addi-tion, for patients with specific needs, a range of design choices are available. Patients with areas of residual ridge resorption, for example, can benefit from the inclusion of materials that compensate for bone loss.

This can help prevent harm to critical structures such as the maxillary sinus and inferior alveolar nerves, located near the implant site. As a result, this approach can overcome the need for complex surgeries such as sinus augmentation when used for implant situations. Stem cells can also be transported on 4D printed implants of tooth-shaped scaffolds, allowing them to develop into genuine teeth. In the case of temporomandibular joints and maxillofacial procedures, 4D printing materials can replace cartilage while undergoing continuous movements to compensate for articulation and occlusion.

8.3   CASE STUDY

A study on 4D-imaging-assisted 4D printing of a dental crown was performed for a canine. Initially, the die-stone models were prepared. Then the stone models were scanned to obtain the surface data. The surface data were exported to different platforms such as Microsoft 3D Builder, Blender, 3D-DOCTOR software, 3Shape dental software, and 3D slicer software for further modifications. In Microsoft 3D Builder, the surface-scanned file of the lower jaw was repaired and saved as an STL file. The repair was made by separating the individual lower mandibular canine tooth (left and right) with the help of a cutting plane. The scanning data processing in 3D Builder software is shown in Figure 8.4.

Similarly, the surface-scanning data of the lower mandible containing incisors and canine teeth were imported to 3D-DOCTOR software for further repair. The file processing in 3D-DOCTOR software is shown in Figure 8.5.

Similarly, the raw surface data of the scanned file was imported into 3D slicer software. The segmentation, angle planes, thickness mapping, texture extension, and reconstruction options were optimized during the file preparation. The scanned data processing in 3D slicer software is shown in Figure 8.6.

The same file was imported into Blender software for modeling. The ZBrush command was used for modification and individual tooth file restoration. The scanned data processed in the Blender software is shown in Figure 8.7.

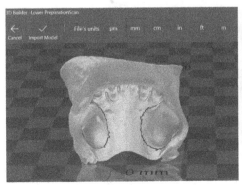 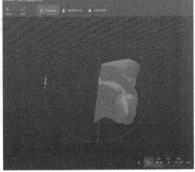

FIGURE 8.4   The coping design in 3D Builder software.

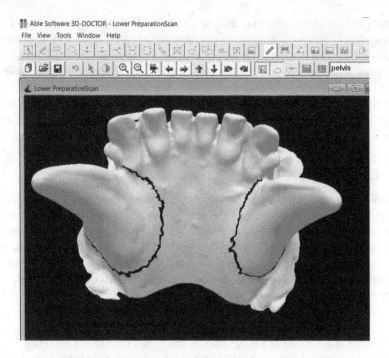

FIGURE 8.5   The coping design in 3D-DOCTOR software.

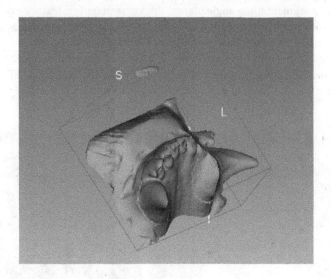

FIGURE 8.6   The coping design in slicer software.

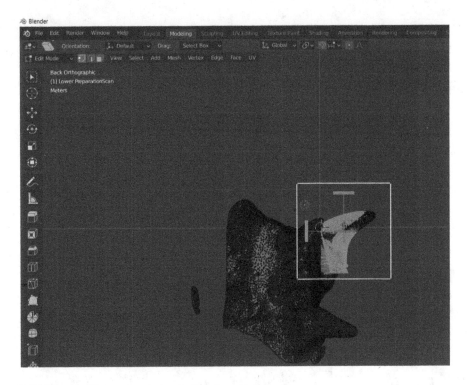

FIGURE 8.7   The coping design in Blender software.

Similarly, the surface-scanned data were processed finally in 3Shape dental software for better visualization and superior modifications. After selecting the region for the crown, the coping was virtually selected over that region and restored by assigning the crown thickness. The coping formation over scanned data in 3Shape dental software is shown in Figure 8.8.

For 4D printing purposes, PVDF-based composites can be prepared by blending with nano-grade materials such as ZnO, barium titanate, and graphene. Similarly, Ni-Ti alloys show prominent results with 4D properties toward solving issues such as dental scaffolds of diabetic patients (hyper and hypoglycemia). The shape-memory alloy-based dental crown fabrication is shown in Figure 8.9.

8.4   SUMMARY

- 4D printing relies on the sequence and path of movements, which determine the self-folding patterns.
- The design should take into account the movement of the circumferential structures around the 4D printed prosthetic appliances.
- Another important aspect is the shaping time under thermal/ physical conditions. The self-folding time can't be infinite; that is, the material should not keep undergoing dynamic changes continuously over time. There should

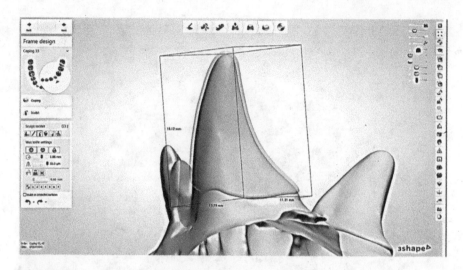

FIGURE 8.8   The coping design in 3Shape dental software.

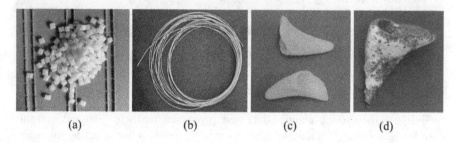

(a)   (b)   (c)   (d)

FIGURE 8.9   (a) PVDF granules, (b) PVDF-matrix-based filament wire, (c) 3D printed dental crown from PVDF-matrix, (d) Ni-Ti alloy-based 3D thermoplastic-pattern-assisted investment casted crown.

   be a so-called self-locking property, which is capable of controlling folding sequences. The application of smart ley-lock connectors will be useful.
   • 4D printed structures will mimic properties of body structure.

4D printing may have a significant impact on all aspects of dentistry. From a further perspective, introduction to smart materials, artificial intelligence, and advanced version of 3D printers may be helpful to obtain smart prosthodontics.

REFERENCES

Aber, J.S., Marzloff, I. and Ries, J., 2010. *Small-Format Aerial Photography: Principles, Techniques and Geoscience Applications.* Amsterdam, the Netherlands: Elsevier.
Akbari, S., Sakhaei, A.H., Kowsari, K., Yang, B., Serjouei, A., Yuanfang, Z. and Ge, Q., 2018. Enhanced multi-material 4D printing with active hinges. *Smart Materials and Structures*, 27(6), p. 065027.

Bruni, A., Serra, F.G., Deregibus, A. and Castroflorio, T., 2019. Shape-memory polymers in dentistry: Systematic review and patent landscape report. *Materials*, 12(14), p. 2216.

Choong, Y.Y.C., Maleksaeedi, S., Eng, H., Wei, J. and Su, P.C., 2017. 4D printing of high-performance shape memory polymer using stereolithography. *Materials and Design*, 126, pp. 219–225.

Cui, H., Miao, S., Esworthy, T., Lee, S.J., Zhou, X., Hann, S.Y., Webster, T.J., Harris, B.T. and Zhang, L.G., 2019. A novel near-infrared light-responsive 4D printed nanoarchitecture with dynamically and remotely controllable transformation. *Nano Research*, 12(6), pp. 1381–1388.

Ge, Q., Dunn, C.K., Qi, H.J. and Dunn, M.L., 2014. Active origami by 4D printing. *Smart Materials and Structures*, 23(9), p. 094007.

Ghazal, A.F., Zhang, M., Mujumdar, A.S. and Ghamry, M., 2022. Progress in 4D/5D/6D printing of foods: Applications and R&D opportunities. *Critical Reviews in Food Science and Nutrition*, pp. 1–24. http://doi.org/10.1080/10408398.2022.2045896.

Hingorani, H., Zhang, Y.F., Zhang, B., Serjouei, A. and Ge, Q., 2019. Modified commercial UV curable elastomers for passive 4D printing. *International Journal of Smart and Nano Materials*, 10(3), pp. 225–236. http://doi.org/10.1080/19475411.2019.1591540.

Hisbergues, M., Vendeville, S. and Vendeville, P., 2009. Zirconia: Established facts and perspectives for a biomaterial in dental implantology. *Journal of Biomedical Materials Research Part B: Applied Biomaterials*, 88(2), pp. 519–529.

Hussein, M.O., 2021. Photogrammetry technology in implant dentistry: A systematic review. *Journal of Prosthetic Dentistry*. https://doi.org/10.1016/j.prosdent.2021.09.015.

Javaid, M. and Haleem, A., 2019. 4D printing applications in medical field: A brief review. *Clinical Epidemiology and Global Health*, 7(3), pp. 317–321.

Khorsandi, D., Fahimipour, A., Abasian, P., Saber, S.S., Seyedi, M., Ghanavati, S., Ahmad, A., De Stephanis, A.A., Taghavinezhaddilami, F., Leonova, A. and Mohammadinejad, R., 2021. 3D and 4D printing in dentistry and maxillofacial surgery: Printing techniques, materials, and applications. *Acta Biomaterialia*, 122, pp. 26–49.

Li, C.H., Wu, C.H. and Lin, C.L., 2020. Design of a patient-specific mandible reconstruction implant with dental prosthesis for metal 3D printing using integrated weighted topology optimization and finite element analysis. *Journal of the Mechanical Behavior of Biomedical Materials*, 105, p. 103700.

Makvandi, P., Ali, G.W., Della Sala, F., Abdel-Fattah, W.I. and Borzacchiello, A., 2019. Biosynthesis and characterization of antibacterial thermosensitive hydrogels based on corn silk extract, hyaluronic acid, and nanosilver for potential wound healing. *Carbohydrate Polymers*, 223, p. 115023.

Makvandi, P., Ali, G.W., Della Sala, F., Abdel-Fattah, W.I. and Borzacchiello, A., 2020. Hyaluronic acid/corn silk extract-based injectable nanocomposite: A biomimetic antibacterial scaffold for bone tissue regeneration. *Materials Science and Engineering: Part C*, 107, p. 110195.

Manouras, T. and Vamvakaki, M., 2017. Field responsive materials: Photo-, electro-, magnetic-and ultrasound-sensitive polymers. *Polymer Chemistry*, 8(1), pp. 74–96.

Pradhan, S.R., Singh, R. and Banwait, S.S., 2020. A-frame work on crown fabrication for veterinary patients using 3D thermoplastic and metal printing. Reference module in materials science and materials. *Engineering*, pp. 1–6. https://doi.org/10.1016/B978-0 -12-820352-1.00063-8.

Pradhan, S.R., Singh, R. and Banwait, S.S., 2022. On 3D printing of dental crowns with direct metal laser sintering for canine. *Journal of Mechanical Science and Technology*, 36. https://doi.org/10.1007/s12206-022-04-y.

Pradhan, S.R., Singh, R., Banwait, S.S., Puhal, M., Singh, S. and Anand, A., 2021a. A comparative study on investment casting of dental crowns for veterinary dentistry by using

ABS patterns with and without wax coating. *E3S Web of Conferences*, 309, pp. 1–6. https://doi.org/10.1051/e3sconf/202130.

Pradhan, S.R., Singh, R. and Banwait, S.S., 2021b. On crown fabrication in prosthetic dentistry of veterinary patients: A review. *Advances in Materials and Processing Technologies*, pp. 1–20. https://doi.org/10.1080/2374068X.2021.1970991.

Pradhan, S.R., Singh, R., Banwait, S.S., Singh, S. and Anand, A., 2021c. 3D printing assisted dental crowns for veterinary patients. *Reference Module in Materials Science and materials Engineering*, 2021, pp. 1–7. Retrieved from http://doi.org/10.1016/B978-0-12 -820352-1.00153-X.

Raja, V. and Fernandes, K.J. (Eds.), 2007. *Reverse Engineering: An Industrial Perspective*. Springer Science & Business Media, Springer: London.

Shirazi, S.F.S., Gharehkhani, S., Mehrali, M., Yarmand, H., Metselaar, H.S.C., Kadri, N.A. and Osman, N.A.A., 2015. A review on powder-based additive manufacturing for tissue engineering: Selective laser sintering and inkjet 3D printing. *Science and Technology of Advanced Materials*, 16(3), p. 033502.

Stansbury, J.W. and Idacavage, M.J., 2016. 3D printing with polymers: Challenges among expanding options and opportunities. *Dental Materials*, 32(1), pp. 54–64.

Subash, A. and Kandasubramanian, B., 2020. 4D printing of shape memory polymers. *European Polymer Journal*, 134, p. 109771.

Sun, W., Starly, B., Daly, A.C., Burdick, J.A., Groll, J., Skeldon, G., Shu, W., Sakai, Y., Shinohara, M., Nishikawa, M. and Jang, J., 2020. The bioprinting roadmap. *Biofabrication*, 12(2), p. 022002.

Vickers, N.J., 2017. Animal communication: When I'm calling you, will you answer too? *Current Biology*, 27(14), pp. R713–R715.

Zambrana, N., Sesma, N., Fomenko, I., Dakir, E.I. and Pieralli, S., 2022. Jaw tracking integration to the virtual patient: A 4D dynamic approach. *Journal of Prosthetic Dentistry*. https://doi.org/10.1016/j.prosdent.2022.02.011.

Zare, E.N., Jamaledin, R., Naserzadeh, P., Afjeh-Dana, E., Ashtari, B., Hosseinzadeh, M., Vecchione, R., Wu, A., Tay, F.R., Borzacchiello, A. and Makvandi, P., 2019. Metal-based nanostructures/PLGA nanocomposites: Antimicrobial activity, cytotoxicity, and their biomedical applications. *ACS Applied Materials and Interfaces*, 12(3), pp. 3279–3300.

Zare, E.N., Lakouraj, M.M., Moghadam, P.N. and Azimi, R., 2013. Novel polyfuran/functionalized multiwalled carbon nanotubes composites with improved conductivity: Chemical synthesis, characterization, and antioxidant activity. *Polymer Composites*, 34(5), pp. 732–739.

Zhou, W., Qiao, Z., Nazarzadeh Zare, E., Huang, J., Zheng, X., Sun, X., Shao, M., Wang, H., Wang, X., Chen, D. and Zheng, J., 2020. 4D-printed dynamic materials in biomedical applications: Chemistry, challenges, and their future perspectives in the clinical sector. *Journal of Medicinal Chemistry*, 63(15), pp. 8003–8024.

9 A Case Study of 4D-Imaging-Assisted 4D Printing for an Efficient Drug-Delivery System for Veterinary Cancer Patients

Vinay Kumar, Nishant Ranjan, Ranvijay Kumar, Ajay Sharma, and Deepika Kathuria

CONTENTS

9.1 INTRODUCTION

In the pharmaceutical field, a few 3D printing technologies are currently being used such as binder jetting, material extrusion (fused deposition modeling (FDM), material jetting, direct powder extrusion (DPE) and semi-solid extrusion (SSE)), selective laser sintering (SLS) (a subcategory of powder bed fusion technology), and vat photo-polymerization (which includes technologies such as continuous liquid interface production (CLIP), digital light processing (DLP), and stereo lithography (SLA)) (Seoane-Viaño et al., 2021; Mohapatra et al., 2022). An individualized object of the desired shape and size can be created with these technologies. Semi-solid extrusion (SSE) is a material extrusion technique based on the deposition of a gel or paste in sequential layers to create a 3D object (Firth et al., 2018). Upon extrusion, the material hardens, allowing the subsequent tiers to be supported by those underneath. The key differences between SSE and other material extrusion techniques, such as FDM or DPE, are in the feedstock materials used (Seoane-Viaño et al., 2021).

DOI: 10.1201/9781003205531-9

In SSE, the starting material is a semi-solid or semi-molten material, whereas in FDM and DPE the printing material is in the form of a solid filament or powder, respectively (Vithani et al., 2019). The literature review, using the Scopus database (of the past 20 years), reveals 1,538 research articles on using 3D printing technology for drug-delivery applications. Based on these studies, Table 9.1 shows the 110 highly investigated key terms such as "wound healing", "3D printed drugs" and "treatment of cancerous cells" that outlined that little work is reported for the treatment of veterinary patients using 3D/4D printing-based drug-delivery systems.

In the literature, SSE is also known as pressure-assisted micro-syringe (PAM) printing, robo-casting or robotic material extrusion, direct ink writing, hydro-gel-forming extrusion, melting extrusion, hot-melt ram extrusion, soft-material extrusion, a melting solidification printing process, cold extrusion-based printing, thermal extrusion, hot-melt pneumatic extrusion, and micro-extrusion (Azad et al., 2020; Nachal et al., 2019; Parhi 2021; de Oliveira et al., 2021). Items can have properties of self-assembly, self-repair, self-disassembly, self-folding, self-sensing, and self-adaptability thanks to the use of smart materials in 4D printing. For example, this cutting-edge technology can create a bone out of stimuli-responsive materials, and this bone will be able to stretch in the human body over time. As a result of the utilization of smart materials and the creation of flexible parts, 4D printing is a revolutionary technology that meets a variety of criteria (Haleem et al., 2021; Raina et al., 2021). The number of studies reported on various key research terms (Table 9.1) indicated that very few researchers have explored the efficient drug-delivery and antioxidant properties of 3D printed polymer-based drugs for veterinary patients. Figure 9.1 show that the past two decades have witnessed a gradual increase in studies related to 3D printed drug-delivery systems for various medical problems such as diabetes, the common cold, influenza, typhoid, etc.

In contrast to 3D printing, 4D printing adds time as a dimension to the created product. 4D printing uses stimuli-responsive materials and printing technologies similar to those used in AM (Lui et al., 2019; Kumar et al., 2022a). To put it another way, 4D printing technology makes use of 3D printers that have been carefully tuned to use stimuli-responsive materials during the layer-by-layer process to meet a variety of continuing needs in various fields (Mallakpour et al., 2022; Kumar et al., 2022b). Smart materials, on the other hand, allow produced items to modify their geometrical shape and function. The advantages of 4D printing technology are numerous (Khoo et al., 2015; Javaid et al., 2022; Kumar et al., 2022c). The highly relevant 110 key terms (Table 9.1) were processed together to obtain the web shown in Figure 9.2 for highlighting the cross-linking of different research areas such as 3D printing, drug preparation, in vitro, in vivo, biocompatible scaffolds, etc. for the development of useful drug-delivery systems for medical applications.

One of the most common uses of 4D bioprinting is in pharmaceutical, bio-adhesion, and drug-delivery systems, in which pharmaceuticals or cells are encapsulated and then released in response to a specific trigger (Malekmohammadi et al., 2021). Researchers must evaluate a variety of elements and domains, including materials, chemical engineering, biomedical engineering, pharmacy, and pathophysiology, to create an appropriate drug-delivery device using 4D printing technology features

TABLE 9.1
Key Terms Investigated for 3D/4D Printed Drug-Delivery Applications by Various Researchers

Id	Term	No. of Studies	Relevance Score
1	Additive manufacturing	7	0.8669
2	Advance	14	0.7652
3	Agent	5	0.8743
4	Article	6	0.5929
5	Assembly	4	1.4844
6	Barrier	6	0.7911
7	Biocompatibility	7	0.5976
8	Biomedical application	8	0.575
9	Biomedical field	4	0.9031
10	Biopolymer	5	1.3441
11	Biosensor	3	1.0922
12	Bone	6	0.7094
13	Bone-tissue engineering	3	0.9492
14	Cancer	4	1.5296
15	Capacity	7	0.6218
16	Cell attachment	3	1.148
17	Characterization	5	0.4951
18	Chitosan	3	1.0907
19	Clinical trial	4	1.4772
20	Combination	5	0.6427
21	Commercialization	3	2.0256
22	Composition	5	0.4443
23	Comprehensive review	3	1.3794
24	Content	6	0.9672
25	Critical role	3	1.2213
26	Current state	3	2.0665
27	Date	4	1.3493
28	Day	5	0.392
29	Delivery	14	0.3982
30	Demand	5	1.4185
31	Detail	4	1.1393
32	Difficulty	3	1.0895
33	Disadvantage	3	1.467
34	Disposal	3	1.3194
35	Drug	8	0.6658
36	Drug release	4	1.2361
37	Energy	7	0.8916
38	Film	5	0.6102
39	Food	6	1.2101
40	Food industry	3	2.2592

(Continued)

TABLE 9.1 (CONTINUED)
Key Terms Investigated for 3D/4D Printed Drug-Delivery Applications by Various Researchers

Id	Term	No. of Studies	Relevance Score
41	Form	7	0.5246
42	Formulation	10	0.5638
43	Future perspective	3	0.9013
44	Gel	5	0.9132
45	Gelatin	3	1.1904
46	Good biocompatibility	3	1.1496
47	Help	3	1.0799
48	Human	4	1.141
49	Human health	4	0.9513
50	Hydrogel	15	0.4025
51	Implementation	4	1.0603
52	Important role	4	1.3013
53	Increase	5	0.8049
54	Industry	8	0.9911
55	Infection	4	1.2439
56	Interest	6	0.7904
57	Layer	4	0.6869
58	Life	5	0.5881
59	Literature	7	0.7623
60	Machine learning	4	1.0595
61	Mechanical property	7	0.5956
62	Medical application	3	0.9446
63	Medical device	3	1.0183
64	Metal	4	0.4649
65	Microfluidic	3	2.2974
66	Microneedle	3	1.7166
67	Morphology	4	1.2384
68	Nanostructure	3	0.7979
69	Nanotechnology	4	1.2541
70	Nature	5	1.4122
71	Need	4	1.0611
72	Next	3	1.6957
73	Number	4	1.289
74	Order	3	1.0431
75	Particle	4	0.8073
76	Patient	7	1.1531
77	Perspective	7	0.6427
78	Poly	4	0.786
79	Possibility	3	1.2885
80	Potential application	3	1.0913

Id	Term	No. of Studies	Relevance Score
81	Preparation	5	0.8999
82	Presence	5	0.7155
83	Printability	5	0.7825
84	Progress	7	0.7157
85	Proliferation	7	0.5723
86	Promising strategy	3	0.9069
87	Recent development	7	0.7585
88	Recent progress	3	0.74
89	Recent year	3	1.8685
90	Regenerative medicine	5	0.6674
91	Release	10	0.5477
92	Safety	6	0.5545
93	Scaffold	9	0.4797
94	Self	5	0.8187
95	Self-healing	4	1.403
96	Sensor	6	0.864
97	Series	3	0.7935
98	Shape	6	0.7658
99	Strain	4	1.0609
100	Surface modification	3	0.6669
101	Temperature	8	0.52
102	Therapeutic agent	3	1.7455
103	Value	6	0.8392
104	Variety	5	0.804
105	View	4	0.9976
106	Vitro	4	0.9953
107	Vitro model	3	1.8431
108	Vivo	3	0.8066
109	Water	8	0.5045
110	Wound healing	3	1.5571

(Shie et al., 2019; Melocchi et al., 2021). The three major paradigms that can be employed in bioprinting for drug administration are: self-regulated, progressive, and immediately triggered. Mirani et al. give an overview of bio-adhesion innovation (Mirani et al., 2017). They demonstrated a multifunctional hydrogel-based smart dressing for wound treatment and diagnosis. It is made up of two main components: pH-responsive sensors and drug-releasing scaffolds (Hosseinzadeh et al., 2019). The main operation of this device is that sensors assess the quantity of infection, and then the medicine is transferred through the scaffolding and injected into the wound. The

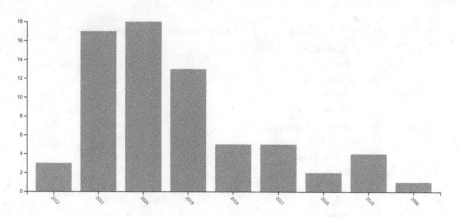

FIGURE 9.1 Number of studies reported on 3D printing-based drug-delivery systems since 2006.

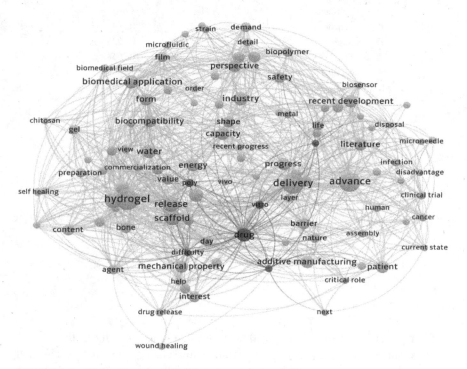

FIGURE 9.2 Web of keywords highlighting the interlinking of research areas: 3D printing and drug-delivery systems.

ability to detect and treat at the same time distinguishes this smart system from standard dressings (Mirani et al., 2017; Shie et al., 2019). Based on Figure 9.2, Figure 9.3 indicates that there is a gap in research and that very little work has been reported on the utilization of 4D imaging integrated 4D capabilities of programmable drugs

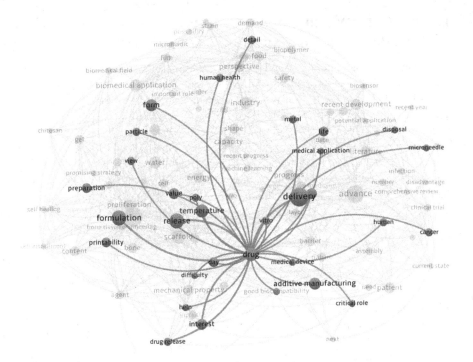

FIGURE 9.3 Research gap for utilization of 4D imaging integrated 4D capabilities of programmable drugs for the development of novel drug-delivery system.

for the development of novel drug-delivery systems for the treatment of cancer cells in veterinary patients.

9.2 RESEARCH GAP

The literature review reveals that, in the past decade, many studies highlighted the role of 3D printing technology in the fabrication of smart and programmable sensors for various biomedical-based 4D printing applications. But, hitherto, much less has been reported on investigating the antioxidant and drug-release capabilities of 3D printable polymer matrix for treating cancerous cells of veterinary patients (mostly in the mouth of bovines and equines). This study reports on investigations performed on the drug-delivery efficiency of medicine-loaded polymer matrix for the 3D/4D printing applications of user-driven drug-delivery systems as a cure for veterinary cancer patients The pilot study performed on drug-release efficiency and the antioxidant properties of polyvinyl alcohol (PVA) polymer matrix loaded with ascorbic acid (as a drug) may be considered as a framework for the preparation of 3D printable (biocompatible polymer matrix) and 4D capable user-driven drugs to treat the cancer cells of veterinary patients with a defined and customizable approach of mouth-cancer treatment.

9.3   CASE STUDY: DRUG-LOADED 3D PRINTED POLYMER FOR TREATMENT OF CANCER CELLS

PVA, one of the biocompatible and biodegradable thermoplastic polymers such as poly lactic acid (PLA) and polyvinylidene fluoride (PVDF), was loaded with ascorbic acid ($C_6H_8O_6$) to investigate the drug release and antioxidant capabilities of PVA-$C_6H_8O_6$ composition/proportion by 4D imaging for 4D printing applications. The initial step was to prepare a 2, 2-diphenyl-1-picrylhydrazyl (DPPH) radical scavenging assay for PVA followed by observation for drug release.

The DPPH radical scavenging power of the loaded drug was evaluated according to the method used by Sharma and Cannoo (2016); 12.4 mg of polymer loaded with the drug was added to 3 ml of methanolic solution of DPPH (0.004%). The various samples were incubated for 30 minutes at room temperature in the dark. Finally, the absorbance was read at 517 nm on a UV-visible spectrophotometer. The percentage inhibition (I %) of DPPH radical was calculated using Equation 9.1:

$$I\%\left[\text{DPPH free radical}\right] = \left[\left(AC - AS\right) / AC\right] \times 100 \quad \text{(Equation 9.1)}$$

Here, AC is the absorbance of the control, and AS is the absorbance of the samples/standard solutions. The percentage inhibition of each sample was evaluated in triplicate.

To evaluate the drug-release potential of the PVA, the polymer block loaded with the drug was put into the fresh double-distilled water in a beaker. After this, a sample was taken from the beaker, and absorbance was noted on a UV-visible spectrophotometer. The same process was repeated after every five minutes, till the constant absorbance on the UV-visible spectrophotometer was obtained. The concentration of the released drug was evaluated with the help of a standard curve of drugs prepared from different standard concentrations. The results obtained for drug release from the PVA sample over time are shown in Table 9.2. Based on Table 9.2, Figure 9.4 outlines the trend of drug release from the PVA-$C_6H_8O_6$ sample. It was observed that the absorbance peak becomes sharper with the passage of time highlighting the increase in the drug-delivery rate. Similarly, the results obtained for antioxidant capabilities of the 3D/4D printable proposed drug are shown in Table 9.3. Equation 9.2 was used to calculate the percentage antioxidant activity of the drug-loaded PVA sample by comparing the absorbance of the test sample with a reference sample called blank:

$$I\%\left[\text{DPPH free radical}\right] = \left[\left(AC - AS\right) / AC\right] \times 100 \quad \text{(Equation 9.2)}$$

The drug release and antioxidant capabilities obtained in PVA-$C_6H_8O_6$ outlined that the novel medicinal applications of such compositions may be used successfully for the fabrication of 3D printed drugs for veterinary cancer patients. By customizing the dosage of $C_6H_8O_6$ in PVA as per the severity/requirement, drug delivery may be executed. Further, the UV-visible spectrophotometer may be used to mimic the 4D imaging of drug release for curing veterinary patients such as bovines and equines.

TABLE 9.2
Drug Release Results for PVA-C$_6$H$_8$O$_6$ Composition (up to 30min)

Wavelength nm	1min	3min	5min	10min	20min	30min
200	0.06	0.137	0.203	0.33	0.462	0.508
202	*0.054*	0.124	0.184	0.299	0.419	0.462
204	*0.048*	0.112	0.167	0.271	0.377	0.419
206	*0.043*	0.103	0.154	0.251	0.345	0.388
208	*0.04*	0.096	0.144	0.236	0.321	0.365
210	0.038	0.092	0.138	0.226	0.304	0.349
212	0.035	0.088	0.134	0.221	0.294	0.34
214	0.034	0.087	0.131	0.218	0.288	0.336
216	0.032	0.086	0.131	0.218	0.288	0.337
218	0.031	0.086	0.132	0.221	0.292	0.342
220	0.031	0.087	0.135	0.228	0.301	0.353
222	0.031	0.09	0.14	0.238	0.315	0.37
224	0.032	0.094	0.147	0.251	0.334	0.392
226	0.033	0.101	0.157	0.269	0.358	0.42
228	0.035	0.109	0.17	0.292	0.388	0.456
230	0.037	0.119	0.186	0.319	0.423	0.498
232	0.041	0.131	0.204	0.35	0.462	0.545
234	0.044	0.144	0.224	0.383	0.505	0.595
236	0.049	0.159	0.247	0.421	0.553	0.652
238	0.055	0.176	0.273	0.462	0.604	0.712
240	0.061	0.196	0.301	0.506	0.658	0.776
242	0.069	0.217	0.332	0.554	0.716	0.844
244	0.077	0.242	0.366	0.606	0.779	0.917
246	0.087	0.269	0.404	0.663	0.845	0.996
248	0.098	0.3	0.446	0.725	0.917	1.078
250	0.11	0.333	0.491	0.789	0.992	1.163
252	0.123	0.367	0.539	0.857	1.067	1.249
254	0.136	0.402	0.586	0.924	1.14	1.332
256	0.149	0.435	0.631	0.986	1.208	1.407
258	0.16	0.465	0.671	1.04	1.265	1.469
260	0.17	0.49	0.703	1.083	1.31	1.516
262	0.177	0.508	0.726	1.113	1.338	1.545
264	0.181	0.518	0.738	1.126	1.349	1.554
266	0.183	0.519	0.739	1.123	1.342	1.545
268	0.18	0.512	0.727	1.103	1.316	1.516
270	0.175	0.495	0.703	1.064	1.271	1.465
272	0.167	0.471	0.667	1.009	1.206	1.395
274	0.156	0.438	0.62	0.939	1.124	1.305
276	0.143	0.4	0.566	0.858	1.029	1.198
278	0.128	0.36	0.509	0.771	0.928	1.083
280	0.114	0.319	0.451	0.684	0.825	0.965

(Continued)

TABLE 9.2 (CONTINUED)
Drug Release Results for PVA-$C_6H_8O_6$ Composition (up to 30min)

Wavelength nm	1min	3min	5min	10min	20min	30min
282	0.1	0.28	0.396	0.601	0.727	0.852
284	0.087	0.243	0.345	0.523	0.634	0.744
286	0.075	0.21	0.297	0.451	0.548	0.644
288	0.065	0.18	0.255	0.388	0.472	0.556
290	0.056	0.155	0.219	0.333	0.406	0.478
292	0.048	0.133	0.188	0.285	0.348	0.41
294	0.042	0.114	0.161	0.244	0.299	0.352
296	0.036	0.099	0.14	0.211	0.259	0.305
298	0.032	0.087	0.122	0.185	0.226	0.267
300	0.029	0.078	0.109	0.164	0.201	0.237
302	0.027	0.071	0.099	0.148	0.181	0.214
304	0.025	0.065	0.091	0.136	0.166	0.196
306	0.024	0.061	0.085	0.126	0.154	0.182
308	0.022	0.058	0.08	0.118	0.145	0.171
310	0.021	0.055	0.076	0.112	0.137	0.161
312	0.021	0.053	0.072	0.106	0.129	0.152
314	0.02	0.05	0.069	0.1	0.122	0.144
316	0.019	0.048	0.066	0.095	0.116	0.135
318	0.018	0.046	0.062	0.09	0.109	0.128
320	0.017	0.044	0.059	0.085	0.103	0.12
322	0.016	0.041	0.056	0.079	0.096	0.112
324	0.016	0.039	0.053	0.075	0.09	0.105
326	0.015	0.037	0.05	0.07	0.085	0.099
328	0.014	0.035	0.047	0.066	0.08	0.093
330	0.013	0.034	0.045	0.063	0.076	0.088
332	0.013	0.033	0.043	0.06	0.073	0.084
334	0.012	0.031	0.042	0.058	0.07	0.081
336	0.012	0.03	0.04	0.056	0.067	0.078
338	0.012	0.03	0.039	0.054	0.065	0.076
340	0.011	0.029	0.038	0.052	0.064	0.073
342	0.01	0.028	0.037	0.051	0.062	0.071
344	0.01	0.027	0.036	0.05	0.061	0.07
346	0.01	0.027	0.035	0.048	0.059	0.068
348	0.009	0.026	0.034	0.047	0.058	0.067
350	0.009	0.025	0.033	0.046	0.056	0.065
352	0.008	0.024	0.032	0.045	0.055	0.063
354	0.008	0.024	0.032	0.043	0.053	0.061
356	0.007	0.023	0.03	0.042	0.051	0.059
358	0.007	0.022	0.029	0.04	0.049	0.057
360	0.007	0.021	0.028	0.038	0.047	0.054
362	0.006	0.02	0.027	0.036	0.045	0.052

Wavelength nm	1min	3min	5min	10min	20min	30min
364	0.006	0.02	0.026	0.034	0.043	0.049
366	0.005	0.019	0.025	0.032	0.04	0.046
368	0.004	0.018	0.023	0.03	0.038	0.043
370	0.003	0.017	0.022	0.028	0.036	0.04
372	0.003	0.016	0.021	0.026	0.033	0.038
374	0.004	0.015	0.02	0.025	0.032	0.036
376	0.003	0.014	0.018	0.024	0.029	0.033
378	0.003	0.013	0.017	0.022	0.028	0.031
380	0.003	0.013	0.016	0.02	0.026	0.029
382	0.002	0.012	0.016	0.019	0.024	0.027
384	0.002	0.011	0.015	0.018	0.023	0.025
386	0.002	0.011	0.014	0.017	0.021	0.024
388	0.002	0.01	0.013	0.015	0.02	0.022
390	0.001	0.01	0.013	0.014	0.019	0.021
392	0.001	0.009	0.012	0.014	0.018	0.019
394	0.001	0.009	0.011	0.013	0.017	0.018
396	0.001	0.009	0.011	0.012	0.016	0.017
398	0	0.008	0.011	0.011	0.015	0.017
400	0	0.008	0.01	0.011	0.014	0.016
402	0	0.008	0.01	0.01	0.014	0.015
404	0	0.008	0.009	0.01	0.013	0.014
406	0	0.007	0.009	0.01	0.013	0.014
408	0	0.007	0.009	0.009	0.013	0.013
410	0	0.007	0.009	0.009	0.012	0.013
412	−0.001	0.007	0.009	0.009	0.012	0.013
414	−0.001	0.007	0.008	0.008	0.011	0.012
416	−0.001	0.007	0.008	0.008	0.011	0.012
418	−0.001	0.007	0.008	0.008	0.011	0.012
420	−0.001	0.006	0.008	0.008	0.011	0.011
422	−0.001	0.006	0.008	0.008	0.011	0.011
424	−0.001	0.006	0.008	0.008	0.011	0.011
426	−0.001	0.006	0.008	0.008	0.011	0.011
428	−0.001	0.006	0.008	0.007	0.01	0.011
430	−0.001	0.006	0.008	0.007	0.01	0.01
432	−0.001	0.006	0.007	0.007	0.01	0.01
434	−0.001	0.006	0.007	0.007	0.01	0.01
436	−0.001	0.006	0.007	0.007	0.01	0.01
438	−0.001	0.006	0.007	0.007	0.01	0.01
440	−0.001	0.006	0.007	0.007	0.01	0.01
442	−0.001	0.006	0.007	0.006	0.009	0.009
444	−0.001	0.006	0.007	0.006	0.009	0.009
446	−0.001	0.006	0.007	0.006	0.009	0.009
448	−0.001	0.006	0.007	0.006	0.009	0.009
450	−0.001	0.006	0.007	0.006	0.009	0.009

(Continued)

TABLE 9.2 (CONTINUED)
Drug Release Results for PVA-$C_6H_8O_6$ Composition (up to 30min)

Wavelength nm	1min	3min	5min	10min	20min	30min
452	−0.001	0.005	0.007	0.006	0.009	0.009
454	−0.001	0.006	0.007	0.006	0.009	0.009
456	−0.001	0.006	0.007	0.006	0.009	0.009
458	−0.001	0.005	0.007	0.006	0.008	0.008
460	−0.001	0.006	0.007	0.006	0.008	0.008
462	−0.001	0.005	0.007	0.006	0.008	0.008
464	−0.001	0.005	0.007	0.006	0.008	0.008
466	−0.001	0.006	0.007	0.006	0.008	0.008
468	−0.001	0.006	0.007	0.006	0.008	0.008
470	−0.001	0.006	0.007	0.006	0.008	0.008
472	−0.001	0.006	0.007	0.006	0.008	0.008
474	−0.001	0.005	0.007	0.006	0.008	0.008
476	−0.001	0.005	0.007	0.006	0.008	0.008
478	−0.001	0.005	0.007	0.006	0.008	0.008
480	−0.001	0.005	0.007	0.006	0.008	0.008
482	−0.001	0.005	0.006	0.006	0.008	0.008
484	−0.001	0.005	0.006	0.006	0.008	0.008
486	−0.001	0.006	0.006	0.005	0.008	0.008
488	−0.001	0.005	0.006	0.005	0.008	0.008
490	−0.001	0.005	0.006	0.005	0.008	0.008
492	−0.001	0.005	0.006	0.005	0.008	0.008
494	−0.001	0.005	0.006	0.005	0.007	0.008
496	−0.001	0.005	0.006	0.005	0.007	0.008
498	−0.001	0.005	0.006	0.005	0.008	0.008
500	−0.001	0.006	0.006	0.005	0.008	0.008
502	−0.001	0.005	0.006	0.005	0.007	0.008
504	−0.001	0.005	0.006	0.005	0.007	0.007
506	−0.001	0.005	0.006	0.005	0.007	0.007
508	−0.001	0.005	0.006	0.005	0.007	0.007
510	−0.001	0.005	0.006	0.005	0.007	0.007
512	−0.001	0.005	0.006	0.005	0.007	0.007
514	−0.001	0.005	0.006	0.005	0.007	0.007
516	−0.001	0.005	0.006	0.005	0.007	0.007
518	−0.001	0.005	0.006	0.005	0.007	0.007
520	−0.001	0.005	0.006	0.005	0.007	0.007
522	−0.001	0.005	0.006	0.005	0.007	0.007
524	−0.001	0.005	0.006	0.005	0.007	0.007
526	−0.001	0.005	0.006	0.004	0.007	0.006
528	−0.001	0.005	0.006	0.004	0.007	0.006
530	−0.001	0.005	0.006	0.004	0.007	0.006
532	−0.001	0.005	0.006	0.004	0.006	0.006

Wavelength nm	1min	3min	5min	10min	20min	30min
534	−0.001	0.005	0.006	0.004	0.006	0.006
536	−0.001	0.005	0.006	0.004	0.006	0.006
538	−0.001	0.005	0.005	0.004	0.006	0.006
540	−0.001	0.005	0.005	0.004	0.006	0.006
542	−0.001	0.005	0.005	0.004	0.006	0.006
544	−0.001	0.004	0.005	0.004	0.006	0.005
546	−0.001	0.004	0.005	0.004	0.006	0.005
548	−0.001	0.004	0.005	0.003	0.006	0.005
550	−0.001	0.004	0.005	0.003	0.005	0.005
552	−0.001	0.004	0.005	0.003	0.005	0.005
554	−0.001	0.004	0.005	0.003	0.005	0.005
556	−0.002	0.004	0.005	0.003	0.005	0.004
558	−0.002	0.004	0.005	0.003	0.005	0.004
560	−0.002	0.004	0.004	0.003	0.005	0.004
562	−0.002	0.004	0.004	0.003	0.005	0.004
564	−0.001	0.004	0.004	0.003	0.004	0.004
566	−0.001	0.004	0.004	0.003	0.005	0.004
568	−0.001	0.004	0.004	0.003	0.004	0.004
570	−0.001	0.004	0.004	0.003	0.004	0.004
572	−0.001	0.004	0.004	0.003	0.004	0.004
574	−0.001	0.004	0.004	0.003	0.004	0.004
576	−0.001	0.004	0.004	0.002	0.004	0.004
578	−0.002	0.003	0.004	0.002	0.004	0.004
580	−0.002	0.004	0.004	0.002	0.004	0.003
582	−0.002	0.004	0.004	0.002	0.004	0.003
584	−0.002	0.004	0.004	0.002	0.004	0.003
586	−0.002	0.003	0.004	0.002	0.004	0.003
588	−0.002	0.003	0.004	0.002	0.003	0.003
590	−0.002	0.003	0.004	0.002	0.003	0.003
592	−0.002	0.003	0.004	0.002	0.003	0.003
594	−0.002	0.003	0.004	0.002	0.003	0.003
596	−0.002	0.003	0.004	0.002	0.003	0.003
598	−0.002	0.003	0.004	0.002	0.003	0.003
600	−0.002	0.003	0.004	0.002	0.003	0.003

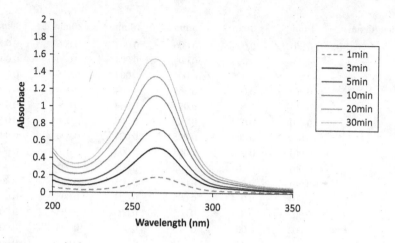

FIGURE 9.4 Absorbance trends obtained under UV spectrophotometer for drug release with time.

TABLE 9.3

Results for Antioxidant Features of PVA-C$_6$H$_8$O$_6$ Composition/Proportion

Replicates	I	II	III	% Antioxidant Activity			Average	S.D.	% Antioxidant Activity
Blank	0.699	0.714	0.722	–	–	–	–	–	–
PLA_12.4	0.305	0.295	0.283	56.36624	58.68347	60.80332	58.61768	2.219275	58.61±2.21

9.4 SUMMARY

The 3D printed polymers, such as PLA, PVA, PVDF, etc., possess various biomedical applications for the fabrication of biocompatible scaffolds and implants. The investigations of drug delivery and antioxidant capabilities for C$_6$H$_8$O$_6$ loaded PVA highlighted that 3D/4D-printing-assisted drug-delivery systems may be successfully incorporated for the treatment of veterinary cancer patients. The drug-loaded (C$_6$H$_8$O$_6$), programmable (4D capable) 3D printed (PVA) medicine-based scaffolds may be used to treat the cancer cells present in the mouth of bovines and equines. 4D imaging supported by a UV-visible spectrophotometer (for evaluation of drug release and antioxidant features) may be used for the treatment of such veterinary cancer patients.

REFERENCES

Azad, M.A., Olawuni, D., Kimbell, G., Badruddoza, A.Z.M., Hossain, M.S. and Sultana, T., 2020. Polymers for extrusion-based 3D printing of pharmaceuticals: A holistic materials–process perspective. *Pharmaceutics*, 12(2), p. 124.

de Oliveira, R.S., Fantaus, S.S., Guillot, A.J., Melero, A. and Beck, R.C.R., 2021. 3D-printed products for topical skin applications: From personalized dressings to drug delivery. *Pharmaceutics*, 13(11), p. 1946.

Firth, J., Basit, A.W. and Gaisford, S., 2018. The role of semi-solid extrusion printing in clinical practice. In A.W. Basit and S. Gaisford (Eds.), *3D Printing of Pharmaceuticals* (pp. 133–151). Cham: Springer.

Haleem, A., Javaid, M., Singh, R.P. and Suman, R., 2021. Significant roles of 4D printing using smart materials in the field of manufacturing. *Advanced Industrial and Engineering Polymer Research*, 4(4), pp. 301–311.

Hosseinzadeh, R., Mirani, B., Pagan, E., Mirzaaghaei, S., Nasimian, A., Kawalec, P., da Silva Rosa, S.C., Hamdi, D., Fernandez, N.P., Toyota, B.D., Gordon, J.W., Ghavami, S. and Akbari, M., 2019. A drug-eluting 3D-printed mesh (GlioMesh) for management of glioblastoma. *Advanced Therapeutics*, 2(11), p. 1900113.

Javaid, M., Haleem, A., Singh, R.P., Rab, S., Suman, R. and Kumar, L., 2022. Significance of 4D printing for dentistry: Materials, process, and potentials. *Journal of Oral Biology and Craniofacial Research*, 12(3), pp. 388–395.

Khoo, Z.X., Teoh, J.E.M., Liu, Y., Chua, C.K., Yang, S., An, J., Leong, K.F. and Yeong, W.Y., 2015. 3D printing of smart materials: A review on recent progress in 4D printing. *Virtual and Physical Prototyping*, 10(3), pp. 103–122.

Kumar, V., Kumar, R., Singh, R. and Kumar, P., 2022a May. On 3D printed biomedical sensors for non-enzymatic glucose sensing applications. *Proceedings of the Institution of Mechanical Engineers, Part H*. https://doi.org/10.1177/09544119221100116.

Kumar, V., Singh, R. and Ahuja, I.P.S., 2022b. Chapter 2. Graphene-reinforced acrylonitrile butadiene styrene composite as smart material for 4D applications. In R. Singh (Ed.), *Additive Manufacturing Materials and Technologies, 4D Printing* (pp. 17–33). Amsterdam: Elsevier. https://doi.org/10.1016/B978-0-12-823725-0.00004-7.

Kumar, V., Singh, R. and Ahuja, I.P.S., 2022c. Chapter 4–3D printed graphene-reinforced polyvinylidene fluoride composite for piezoelectric properties. In R. Singh (Ed.), *Additive Manufacturing Materials and Technologies, 4D Printing* (pp. 51–66). Amsterdam: Elsevier. https://doi.org/10.1016/B978-0-12-823725-0.00009-6.

Lui, Y.S., Sow, W.T., Tan, L.P., Wu, Y., Lai, Y. and Li, H., 2019. 4D printing and stimuli-responsive materials in biomedical aspects. *Acta Biomaterialia*, 92, pp. 19–36.

Malekmohammadi, S., Sedghi Aminabad, N., Sabzi, A., Zarebkohan, A., Razavi, M., Vosough, M., Bodaghi, M. and Maleki, H., 2021. Smart and biomimetic 3D and 4D printed composite hydrogels: Opportunities for different biomedical applications. *Biomedicines*, 9(11), p. 1537.

Mallakpour, S., Tabesh, F. and Hussain, C.M., 2022 March. A new trend of using poly (vinyl alcohol) in 3D and 4D printing technologies: Process and applications. *Advances in Colloid and Interface Science*, 301, p. 102605.

Melocchi, A., Uboldi, M., Cerea, M., Foppoli, A., Maroni, A., Moutaharrik, S., Palugan, L., Zema, L. and Gazzaniga, A., 2021. Shape memory materials and 4D printing in pharmaceutics. *Advanced Drug Delivery Reviews*, 173, pp. 216–237.

Mirani, B., Pagan, E., Currie, B., Siddiqui, M.A., Hosseinzadeh, R., Mostafalu, P., Zhang, Y.S., Ghahary, A. and Akbari, M., 2017. An advanced multifunctional hydrogel-based dressing for wound monitoring and drug delivery. *Advanced Healthcare Materials*, 6(19), p. 1700718.

Mohapatra, S., Kar, R.K., Biswal, P.K. and Bindhani, S., 2022. Approaches of 3D printing in current drug delivery. *Sensors International*, 3, p. 100146.

Nachal, N., Moses, J.A., Karthik, P. and Anandharamakrishnan, C., 2019. Applications of 3D printing in food processing. *Food Engineering Reviews*, 11(3), pp. 123–141.

Parhi, R., 2021. A review of three-dimensional printing for pharmaceutical applications: Quality control, risk assessment, and future perspectives. *Journal of Drug Delivery Science and Technology*, 64, p. 102571.

Raina, A., Haq, M.I.U., Javaid, M., Rab, S. and Haleem, A., 2021. 4D printing for automotive industry applications. *Journal of the Institution of Engineers (India): Series D*, 102(2), pp. 521–529.

Seoane-Viaño, I., Trenfield, S.J., Basit, A.W. and Goyanes, A., 2021. Translating 3D printed pharmaceuticals: From hype to real-world clinical applications. *Advanced Drug Delivery Reviews*, 174, pp. 553–575.

Sharma, A. and Cannoo, D.S., 2016. Effect of extraction solvents/techniques on polyphenolic contents and antioxidant potential of the aerial parts of Nepeta leucophylla and the analysis of their phytoconstituents using RP-HPLC-DAD and GC-MS. *RSC Advances*, 6(81), pp. 78151–78160.

Shie, M.Y., Shen, Y.F., Astuti, S.D., Lee, A.K.X., Lin, S.H., Dwijaksara, N.L.B. and Chen, Y.W., 2019. Review of polymeric materials in 4D printing biomedical applications. *Polymers*, 11(11), p. 1864.

Vithani, K., Goyanes, A., Jannin, V., Basit, A.W., Gaisford, S. and Boyd, B.J., 2019. An overview of 3D printing technologies for soft materials and potential opportunities for lipid-based drug delivery systems. *Pharmaceutical Research*, 36(1), pp. 1–20.

Index

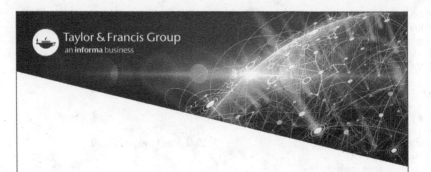